The 5:2 Diet Cookbook

120 Easy and Delicious Recipes for Your Two Days of Fasting

Edited by Laura Herring, Photographs by William Reavell

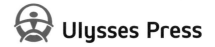
Ulysses Press

Text and photography © Ebury Press 2013. All rights reserved. No part of this publication may be reproduced, stored in a retrieval system, or transmitted in any form or by any means, electronic, mechanical, photocopying, recording or otherwise, without the prior permission of the copyright owner.

Published in the US by
ULYSSES PRESS
PO Box 3440
Berkeley, CA 94703
www.ulyssespress.com

ISBN 978-1-61243-282-3
Library of Congresss Conrol Number: 2013943005

First published in 2013 in the UK as *The Fasting Day Cookbook* by Ebury Press, an imprint of Ebury Publishing, A Random House Group Company

Printed in the United States by Bang Printing

10 9 8 7 6 5 4 3 2 1

Design by Seagull Design
Photography by William Reavell
Project editor: Laura Herring
Food stylist: Emma Marsden
Props stylist: Jo Harris
Consultant dietician: Fiona Hinton
US acquisitions: Kelly Reed
US editor: Lauren Harrison
US proofreader: Elyce Berrigan-Dunlop
Cover design: Michelle Thompson | Fold & Gather Design

Distributed by Publishers Group West

contents

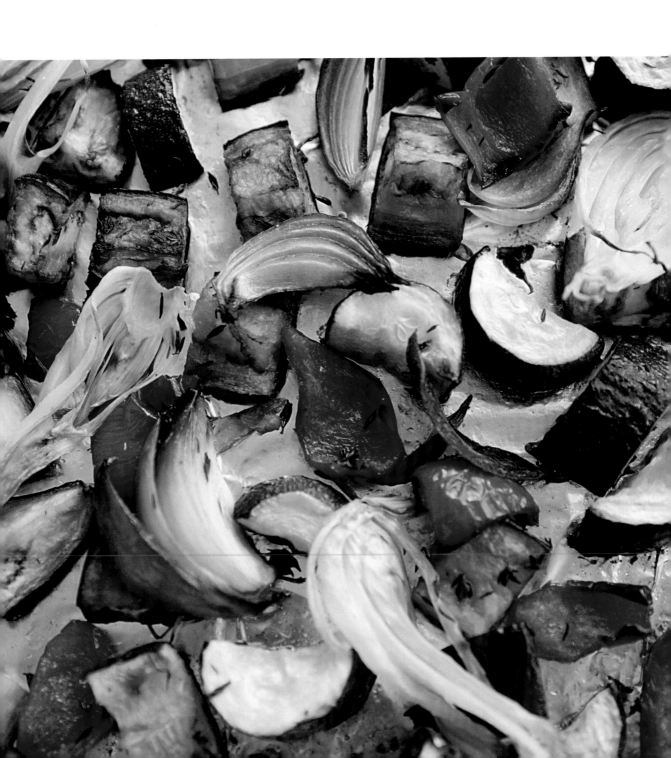

introduction

There is much evidence associating low-calorie diets with many long-term health benefits. A restricted diet is thought to reduce our risk of developing serious illnesses like diabetes and cancer, and to help us live for longer. It is not altogether reasonable, however, to expect people to follow a continuously reduced-calorie diet, and more commonly it is recommended to include two low-calorie days each week, while eating normally the remainder of the time. On fast days, women should consume no more than 500 calories, and men, no more than 600 calories.

During their fast days, many people choose to follow a traditional three-meals-a-day routine, with a low-calorie breakfast, lunch and dinner. Others prefer a light start to the day, saving up their calories for a hearty meal in the evening. Alternatively, you could start the day with a larger breakfast, eating just very small meals for the rest of the day. As long as you stay within your calories, you can mix-and-match in whatever way suits you best. *The 5:2 Diet Cookbook* allows you to do just this, with a delicious range of simple recipes for breakfast, lunch and dinner—and even a chapter on snacks and drinks—all of which you can eat, guilt-free, on your fasting days. Each recipe includes a total calorie count at the top of the page and the calorie brackets are color-coded for ease of use (see the table on page 8) so that you can plan out your

day—there are also some suggested meal plans on pages 180–7 covering a range of calorie limits.

Following a diet doesn't mean you have to miss out on all your favorite foods. In fact, flavor and variety are what will stop you from feeling like you're on a diet at all. The recipes in this book make use of many slow-release energizers like oats, beans and lentils to help you feel fuller for longer, drawing inspiration from all kinds of cuisine, including Chinese, Indian, Thai and Italian. Start the day with a cranberry Morning Muffin (page 19), Huevos Rancheros (page 22) or a Low-cal Eggs and Bacon (page 32). Enjoy a midday meal of Grilled Jumbo Prawns with Chili Soy Sauce (page 45) or Fattoush (page 53), and end your day with well-deserved Minted Lamb (page 116), Chicken with Herby Nut Stuffing (page 127) or Lamb and Bamboo Shoot Red Curry (page 135). There is a wide variety to pick from, so you can eat different, exciting meals on every fast day.

For many dieters, snacking is a hard habit to break. *The 5:2 Diet Cookbook* has this covered too. With ideas from as low as 40 calories, choose from an irresistible range of snacks to see you through the day: Saffron Scones (page 159), Oaty Fruit Bites (page 160) or for when chocolate is the only answer, a luxurious Rich and Dark Spiced Hot Chocolate (page 163).

One of the main complaints when following a new eating plan is the amount of preparation involved, or the inconvenience of providing for other family members at mealtimes. Many of the recipes in *The 5:2 Diet Cookbook* are designed to serve four or more, meaning you can supplement them with extra side dishes to provide a filling meal for the rest of the family. Many other recipes are suitable for making in larger batches and freezing for upcoming diet days.

With such a tempting range of meals and snacks to choose from, you'll be able to eat just as well on your fast days as on your feast days!

Color-Coded Calories

Using the easy-to-follow colored stripes at the top of each recipe you can plan your daily intake at a glance. Each recipe also includes an exact calorie count.

- 0–100 calories per serving

- 101–200 calories per serving

- 201–300 calories per serving

- 301–400 calories per serving

- 401–500 calories per serving

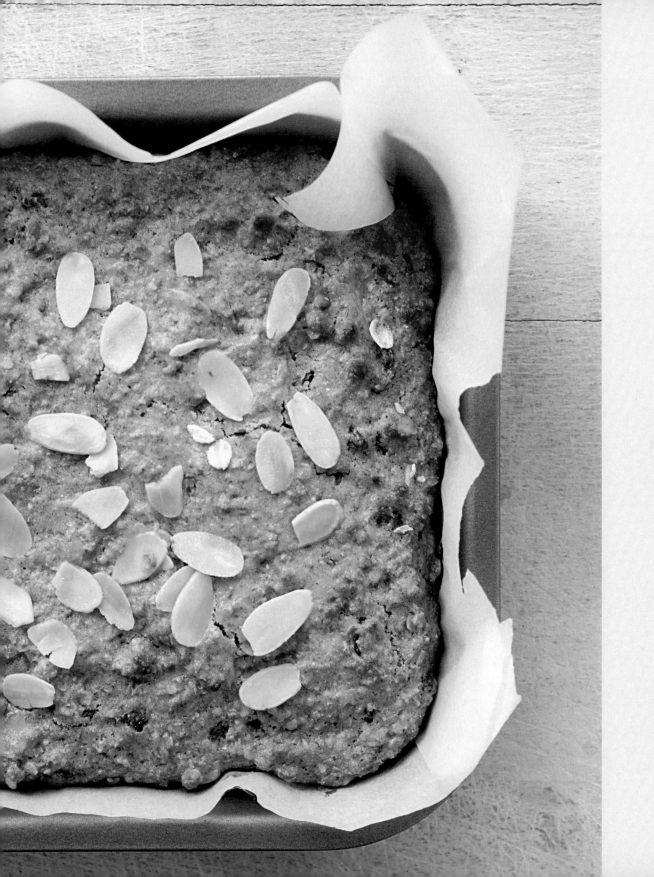

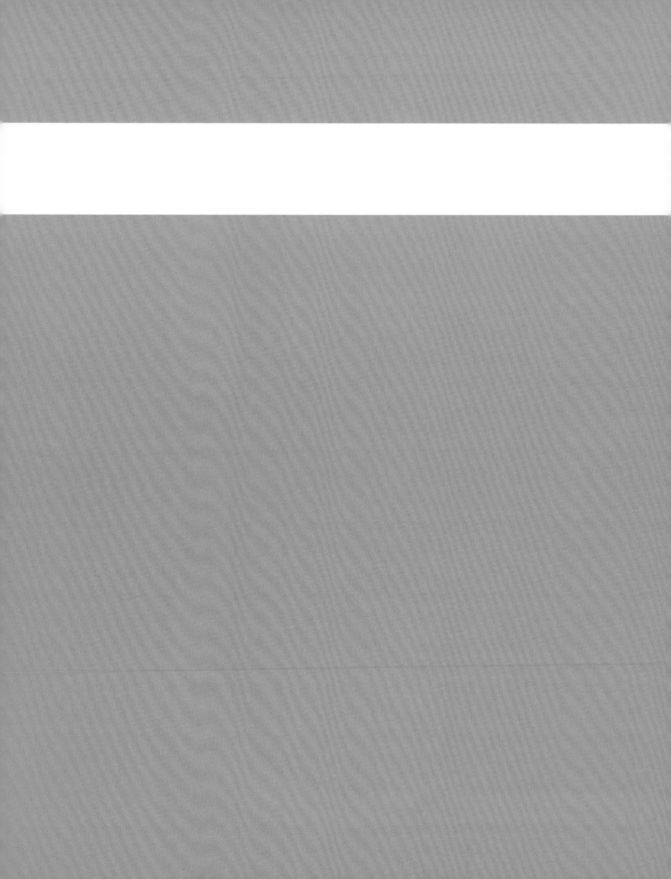

breakfast

Chilled Melon and Ginger Salad

CALORIES PER SERVING: 105

Serves 4 | Preparation time: 15 minutes, plus chilling time | Cooking time: 10 minutes

This simple summer salad features the winning combination of melon and ginger. Here the mellow colors of several different melons blend together beautifully to make a very pretty dish.

1 small charentais or
    cantaloupe melon
1 small galia melon
½ large honeydew
    melon
12oz (350g) watermelon

for the dressing
2 tbsp baker's sugar
1 tbsp chopped
    preserved stem
    ginger in syrup,
    drained
2 tbsp orange juice
2 tsp lemon juice

First make the dressing. Place the sugar and ginger in a small saucepan with ½ cup (120ml) water. Heat gently to dissolve the sugar, then bring to a boil and simmer for 10 minutes.

Transfer to a bowl and stir in the orange and lemon juices. Set aside to cool.

Peel each melon and discard the seeds. Cut the flesh into thin wedges and mix together in a large bowl.

Pour the cooled dressing on top, stir well, cover and chill for 1 hour before serving.

Melon with Summer Fruits

CALORIES PER SERVING: 112

Serves 4 | Preparation time: 20 minutes, plus resting time

Cubes of scented, pale green and orange melon are tossed with red summer fruits in an orange, melon sauce to make a delightful fruit salad. Choose melons that are very ripe. A ripe melon should give slightly when you apply pressure at the stem end.

½ galia melon
1 charentais or
   cantaloupe melon
5oz (150ml) freshly
   squeezed orange
   juice
¼lb (125g) strawberries
½lb (225g) raspberries
4 tbsp fat-free Greek-
   style yogurt
4 tsp honey

Cut the melons into thick wedges, then scoop out the seeds and remove the skin using a sharp knife. Cut the galia melon and half of the charentais or cantaloupe melon into cubes and place in a serving bowl.

Roughly chop the remaining charentais or cantaloupe melon and place in a blender with the orange juice. Process until smooth and then pour over the melon cubes.

Halve or quarter the strawberries, depending on their size, and add to the melon with the raspberries. Leave at room temperature for at least half an hour to allow the flavors to mingle before serving.

Serve with the Greek-style yogurt and honey.

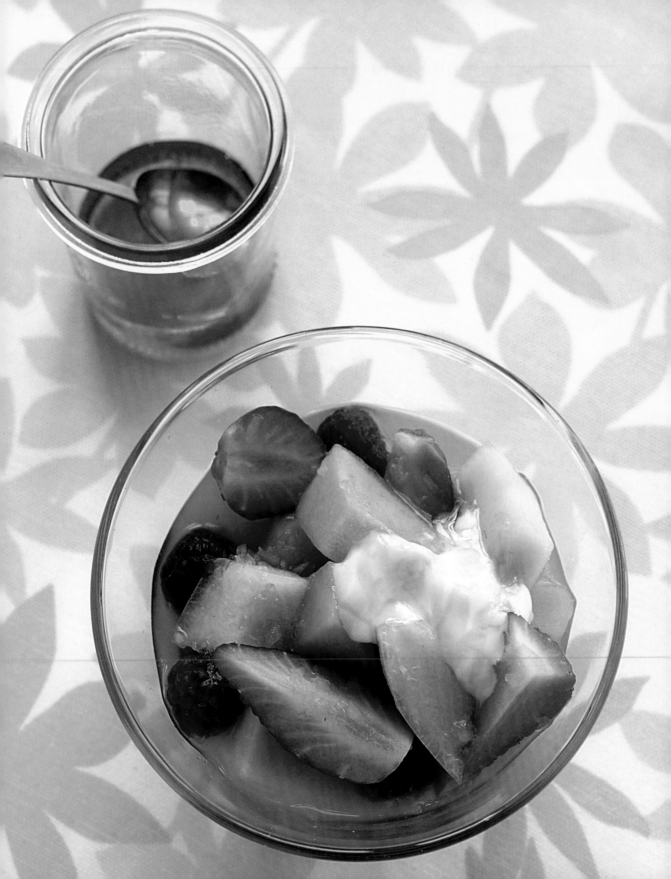

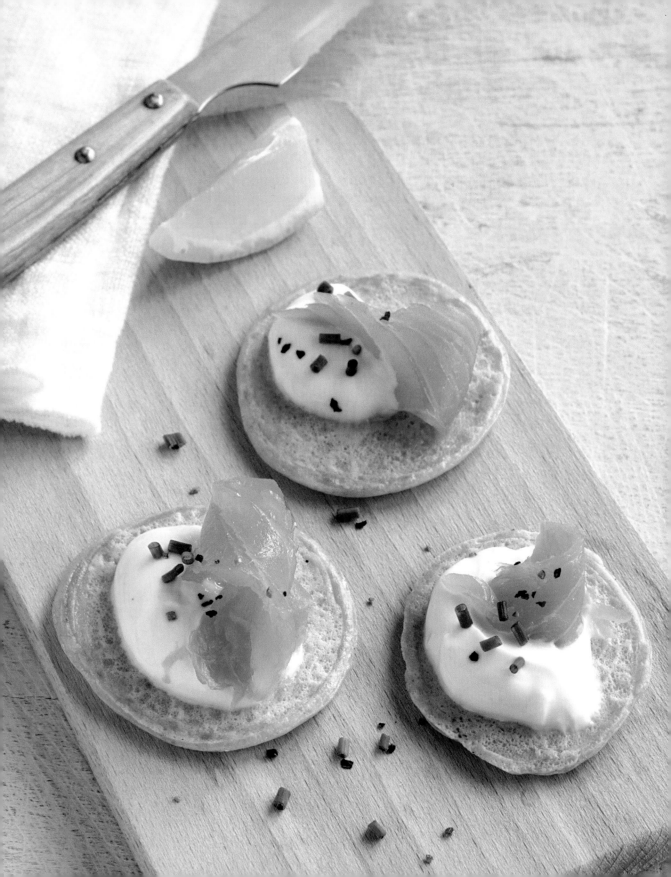

Mini Pancakes with Smoked Salmon

CALORIES PER SERVING: 136

Serves 2 | Preparation time: 10 minutes | Cooking time: 5 minutes

Smoked salmon always seems like such a treat. Served this way, it is filling and satisfying. The cool dressing, creamy salmon and hot pancakes make a luxurious breakfast.

2 tbsp cream cheese
a squeeze of lemon
    juice
1oz (25g) smoked
    salmon
2 tsp chopped chives
salt and pepper

for the pancakes
¼c plus 2½ tbsp (50g)
    all-purpose flour
1 medium egg
2 tbsp low-fat milk
4–6 sprays low-cal
    cooking spray
salt and white pepper

To make the pancakes, sift the flour into a bowl and season with the salt and white pepper. Make a well in the middle, crack in the egg and add the milk and 3½ tablespoons (50ml) water. Whisk the ingredients together briskly until combined.

Heat a non-stick frying pan over a medium heat and spray with the cooking spray. Place three large spoonfuls (half the mixture), well spaced apart, in the pan. Cook until bubbles appear on the surface and then flip the pancakes over and cook on the other side for a minute or two, until golden. Keep the pancakes warm under a piece of foil while you repeat with the rest of the batter.

Beat the cream cheese with the lemon juice, and season with salt and pepper to taste. Place three pancakes on each plate and top each with the cream cheese mixture and the smoked salmon. Sprinkle with the chives.

Wholesome Oatmeal with Cinnamon

CALORIES PER SERVING: 137

Serves 1 | Preparation time: 5 minutes | Cooking time: 15 minutes

A traditional oatmeal breakfast has been given a delicious and healthy boost in this recipe. This warming dish will keep you going until lunch.

2 tbsp (20g) rolled oats
1 tsp mixed seeds,
   such as pumpkin,
   sunflower, sesame
   and poppy
8 golden raisins
2 tbsp low-fat plain
   yogurt
a pinch of cinnamon

Put the oats in a small pan. Add the seeds and raisins and ½ cup (130ml) water. Bring to a boil and simmer for 5–10 minutes, until the water has been completely absorbed by the oats and the oatmeal is thick.

Spoon into a bowl, top with the yogurt and sprinkle with the cinnamon.

Fruit and Yogurt Parfait

CALORIES PER SERVING: 164

Serves 1 | Preparation time: 5 minutes | Cooking time: 2 minutes

A lovely, creamy and fruity start to the day. Use a combination of whatever fruits are in season and experiment with different varieties.

1 tbsp rolled oats
1 tsp golden baker's
   sugar
¼ tsp pumpkin pie spice
1 tsp slivered almonds
3.5oz (100g) fruit (use
   either chopped hard
   fruit or soft fruits)
3.5oz (100g) low-fat
   plain yogurt

Put the oats, sugar, pumpkin pie spice and almonds in a pan and heat for a couple of minutes until the almonds have turned golden and the sugar has dissolved and starts to stick all the ingredients together.

Spoon half the fruit into a glass, top with half the yogurt, then half the oat mixture. Repeat to make another layer, then serve.

Scones with Blueberries

CALORIES PER SERVING: 168

Makes 10 | Preparation time: 10 minutes | Cooking time: 15–20 minutes

These lightly spiced scones are pan-fried to give a soft, spongy texture on the inside and a sweet, crisp crust. Once fried, they're topped with fresh blueberries and lightly grilled to bring out the full-scented flavor of the berries.

1⅓c (175g) self-rising
   whole wheat flour
a pinch of salt
1 tsp baking powder
¼ tsp ground mace
¼ tsp ground cloves
5 tbsp unsalted butter
2½ tbsp (25g) rice flour
2 tbsp baker's sugar
3 tbsp low-fat milk
2 tbsp vegetable oil
½lb (225g) blueberries
1 tbsp powdered sugar

Sift the flour, salt, baking powder, mace and cloves into a bowl. Add 3½ tablespoons (50g) of the butter, cut into small pieces, and rub in using your fingertips until the mixture resembles fine breadcrumbs. Stir in the rice flour and baker's sugar. Add the milk and mix until it forms a fairly soft dough, using a pastry cutter.

Turn the dough out on to a lightly floured surface and knead very gently. Cut into 10 even-sized pieces. Using lightly floured hands, shape each piece into a small, flat scone.

Melt 1 tablespoon (15g) of the remaining butter with half the oil in a large heavy-based frying pan or griddle. Place half of the scones in the pan and fry gently over a medium-low heat for 3–4 minutes until golden underneath. Turn the scones over and cook for another 3–4 minutes until cooked through. Transfer to a large baking sheet. Melt the remaining butter with the oil and fry the rest of the scones.

Preheat the grill to medium. Spoon the blueberries on to the scones, piling them up slightly in the center. Sprinkle with the powdered sugar. Place under the grill for about 2 minutes, watching closely, until the blueberries are bubbling and the scone edges are lightly toasted. Serve immediately.

Note: It is essential to cook the scones over a very gentle heat. A high temperature will overcook the crusts while the centers remain raw.

Morning Muffins

CALORIES PER SERVING: 175

Makes 12 │ Preparation time: 15 minutes │ Cooking time: 20 minutes

Moist muffins bursting with cranberries almost taste a little festive. Have all the dry ingredients mixed together, and prepare the muffin tin the night before. Serve straight from the oven—these muffins do not reheat well.

6oz (175g) fresh
   cranberries
½c (50g) powdered
   sugar, sifted
1¼c (150g) whole wheat
   flour
1¼c (150g) all-purpose
   flour
1 tbsp baking powder
1 tsp pumpkin pie spice
½ tsp salt
½c (50g) soft light
   brown sugar
1 medium egg
1c (250ml) low-fat milk
¼c (60ml) vegetable oil

Halve the cranberries and place in a bowl with the powdered sugar. Toss gently to mix.

Line a 12-cup muffin tin with paper liners or simply grease with butter. Sift together the flours, baking powder, pumpkin pie spice, salt and brown sugar in a large bowl. Make a well in the center.

Preheat the oven to 350˚F/180˚C. Beat the egg with the milk and oil. Add to the dry ingredients and stir just until blended, then lightly and quickly stir in the cranberries. The mixture should look roughly mixed, with lumps and floury pockets.

Fill the muffin cups two-thirds full with the mixture. Bake in the oven for about 20 minutes or until well risen and golden brown.

Transfer the muffins to a wire rack to cool slightly. Serve while still warm.

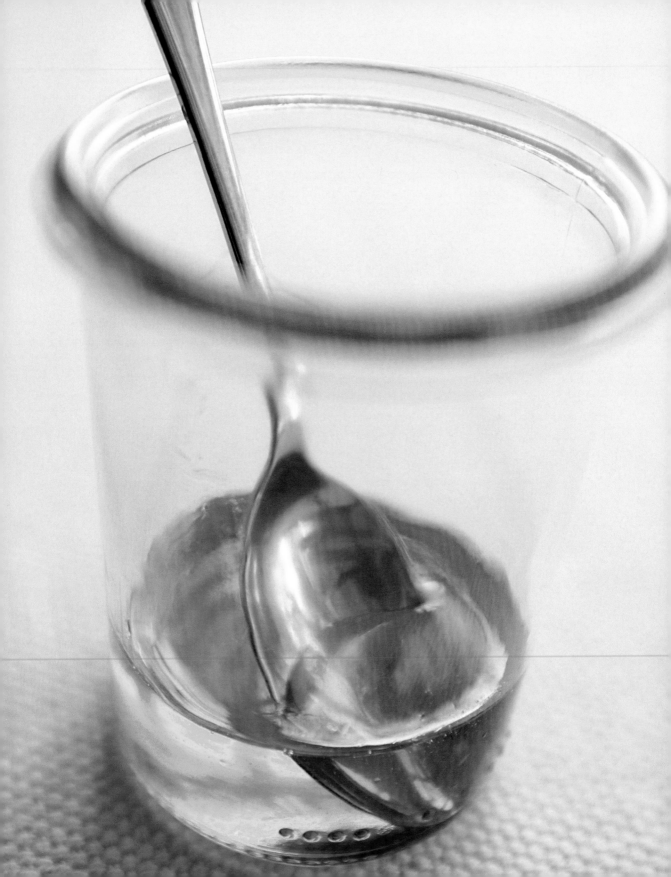

Honey and Yogurt Muffins

CALORIES PER SERVING: 180

Makes 12 | Preparation time: 15 minutes | Cooking time: 20 minutes

These home-style muffins have a lovely subtle spice. They also freeze well.

2c (225g) all-purpose flour
1½ tsp baking powder
1 tsp baking soda
a pinch of salt
½ tsp ground pumpkin pie spice
¼ tsp ground nutmeg
¼c plus 1 tbsp (50g) medium
    oatmeal, plus extra for
    dusting
¼c (50g) light muscovado sugar
3½ tbsp (50g) butter
½lb (225g) Greek-style yogurt
½c (125ml) milk
1 medium egg
4 tbsp honey

Preheat the oven to 400˚F/200˚C. Line a twelve-cup muffin tin with paper liners or simply grease with butter. Sift the flour, baking powder, baking soda, salt, pumpkin pie spice and nutmeg into a bowl. Stir in the oatmeal and sugar.

Melt the butter and leave to cool slightly. Mix the yogurt and milk together in a bowl, then beat in the egg, butter and honey. Pour over the dry ingredients and stir in quickly until just blended.

Divide the mixture equally among the muffin cups. Sprinkle with oatmeal and bake for about 20 minutes, until well risen and just firm to the touch. Remove from the oven and leave in the tins for 5 minutes, then transfer to a wire rack.

Breakfast Smoothie

CALORIES PER SERVING: 190

Serves 1 | Preparation time: 5 minutes

Oats will help you stay fuller for longer and this rich, creamy smoothie tastes truly decadent.

½ banana, chopped
2 tbsp rolled oats
2.5oz (75ml) low-fat
    plain yogurt
¼c plus 1 tbsp (75ml)
    non-fat milk
2oz (50g) frozen berries

Put the banana pieces in a blender. Add the oats, yogurt, milk and frozen berries and blend the mixture until smooth, then pour into a glass and serve.

Huevos Rancheros

CALORIES PER SERVING: 204

Serves 2 | Preparation time: 5 minutes | Cooking time: 20 minutes

This Mexican-inspired breakfast has a spicy kick to get your day started. You can serve this in one large dish or individual ramekins.

1 tsp olive oil
2 spring onions, chopped
½ red pepper, chopped
½ red chile pepper, finely chopped
1 (8-ounce) can of chopped tomatoes
1 tsp balsamic vinegar
2 medium eggs
1 whole wheat pita bread
1 tbsp flat-leaf parsley or cilantro, roughly chopped
salt and pepper

Heat the oil in a frying pan and fry the spring onions, red pepper and chile for about 5 minutes, until softened and golden.

Add the chopped tomatoes and vinegar and season well with salt and pepper. Bring to a boil and simmer for a couple of minutes, until thickened.

Make two wells in the middle of the pan and crack an egg into each. Cook until the whites have started to set, then cover and continue to cook until the white is completely cooked through.

Meanwhile, cut the pita bread into triangles and toast lightly.

Divide the huevos rancheros between two plates and serve with a sprinkle of parsley or cilantro and the toasted pita.

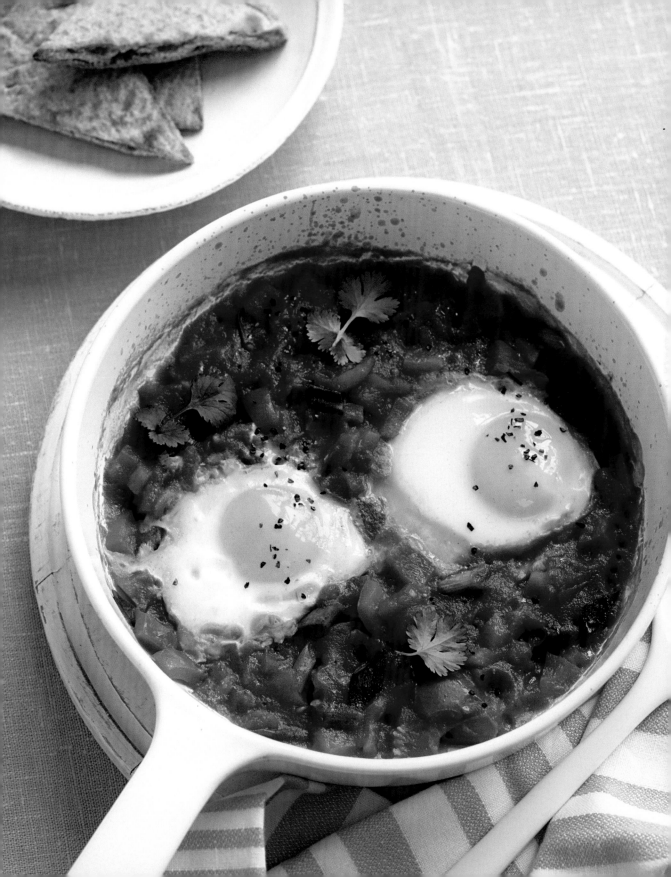

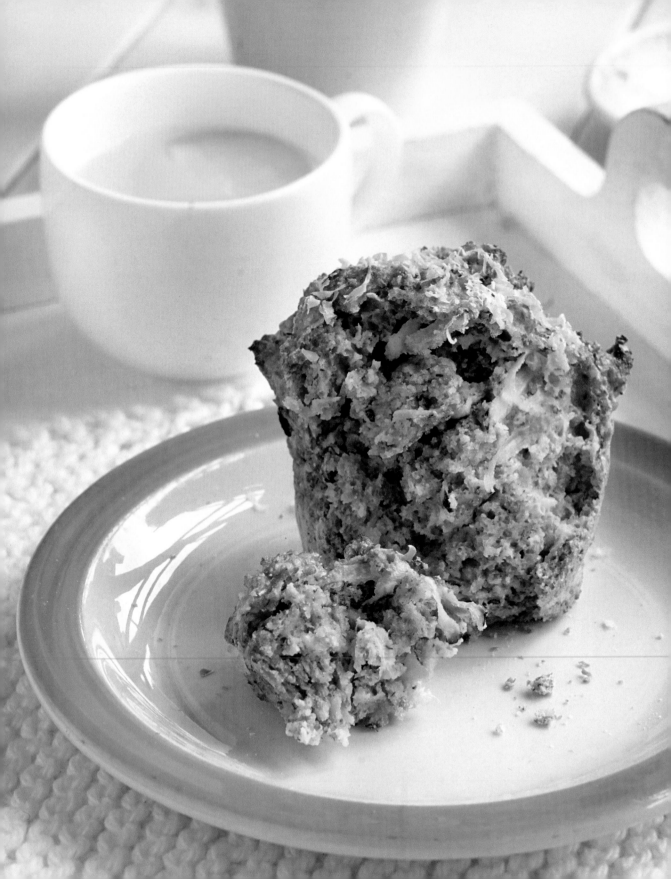

Savory Muffins

CALORIES PER SERVING: 215

Makes 6 | Preparation time: 15 minutes | Cooking time: 25–30 minutes

These may sound a bit strange for breakfast but they really hit the spot. These also store well; once cool, wrap in plastic wrap and freeze for up to a month.

1 medium zucchini,
   around 6oz (175g),
   grated
1 medium carrot, around
   4oz (125g), grated
2c (250g) self-rising
   whole wheat flour
1.5oz (40g) pecorino
   cheese, grated
a pinch of salt
½ tsp ground white
   pepper
6oz (175g) low-fat plain
   yogurt
3½ tbsp (50ml) low-fat
   milk
2 medium eggs

Preheat the oven to 400˚F/200˚C. Put the grated zucchini and carrot in a large bowl. Add the flour, cheese, salt and pepper and toss roughly to mix everything together.

In a separate bowl, beat the yogurt, milk and eggs. Make a well in the center of the flour mixture and pour in the yogurt mixture. Roughly combine all the ingredients together. Don't worry if there are still some floury patches; these will cook out once the muffins are baked.

Line a six-cup muffin tin with paper liners or simply grease with butter. Divide the mixture among the muffin cups and bake for 25–30 minutes, until a skewer pushed into the middle comes out clean.

Remove from the tin and cool on a wire rack until just warm, then serve.

Prosciutto, Melon and Ricotta Salad

CALORIES PER SERVING: 228

Serves 4 | Preparation time: 15 minutes, plus chilling time

Inspired by flavors now synonymous with Italian cuisine, this is a particularly fresh-tasting salad that makes a surprisingly good breakfast.

5oz (150g) ricotta
    cheese
2 tbsp chopped mixed
    fresh herbs, such as
    chervil, chives and
    basil
½ tsp lemon juice
1 small cantaloupe or
    charentais melon
¼lb (125g) prosciutto
12 black olives, pitted
2oz (50g) watercress
    leaves
salt and pepper
grated lemon zest, to
    garnish

for the dressing
1 small ripe tomato
1 small shallot, peeled
1 small garlic clove,
    crushed
1 tsp grated lemon zest
1 tsp lemon juice
½ tbsp red wine vinegar
3 tbsp extra virgin olive oil

In a small bowl, beat the ricotta with the herbs, lemon juice and salt and pepper, to taste. Cover and chill for 30 minutes.

Meanwhile, prepare the dressing. Skin (see page 53), deseed and dice the tomato. Finely chop the shallot. Place all of the dressing ingredients in a small bowl and stir to combine. Season, to taste, with salt and pepper. Set aside until required.

Just before serving, cut the melon into wedges and scoop out the seeds. Peel and slice again into thin wedges.

Divide the melon slices among individual serving plates and top with the prosciutto, olives and watercress leaves. Top each salad with the ricotta.

Spoon the dressing on top and garnish with lemon zest.

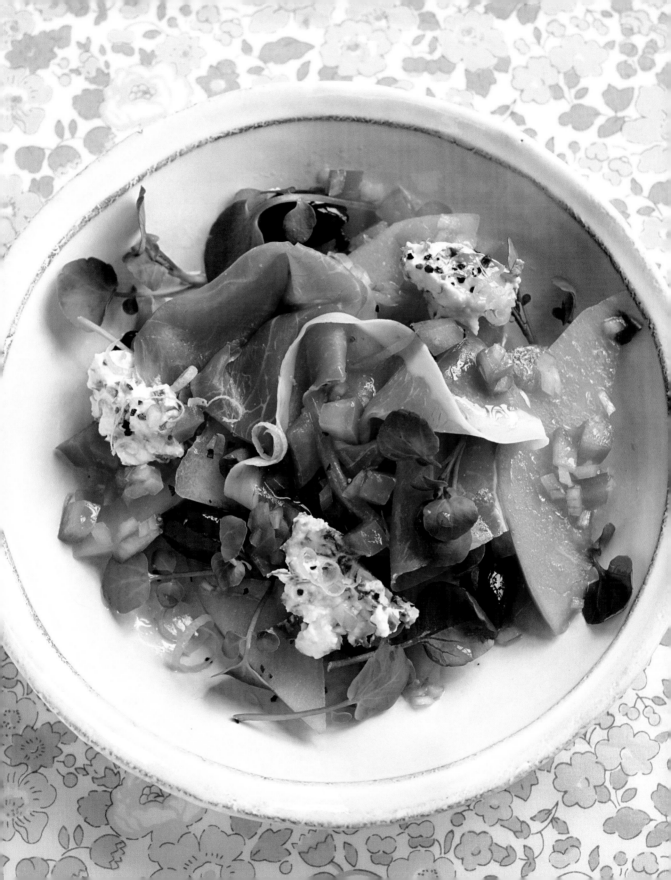

Poached Egg, Florentine-Style

CALORIES PER SERVING: 244

Serves 1 │ Preparation time: 5 minutes │ Cooking time: 20 minutes

A classic pairing of eggs and spinach, minus the rich sauce. This has a great combination of flavors and will keep hunger at bay.

1 tsp butter
1 tomato, deseeded and
    diced
a large handful of
    spinach
1 medium egg
½ English muffin
1 tbsp freshly grated
    Parmesan cheese
salt and pepper

Heat the butter in a pan and add the tomato and spinach. Season well with salt and pepper. Cook for a couple of minutes, until the spinach has just wilted.

Bring a small pan of water to a boil. Stir the water with a spoon to create a swirl, then crack the egg into a small bowl and slide the egg into the middle of the swirl. Poach for 3–4 minutes until the white is firm and opaque.

Toast the muffin and place on a plate. Spoon the spinach and tomato mixture on top. Using a slotted spoon, lift the poached egg out of the water and drain on a paper towel. Place on top of the spinach mixture and sprinkle with the Parmesan. Season well and serve.

Eggs with Smoked Salmon

CALORIES PER SERVING: 249

Serves 4 | Preparation time: 5 minutes | Cooking time: 3–5 minutes

This can be made in the time it takes to boil an egg. It's best if the crème fraîche is at room temperature when you use it.

4 medium eggs
3.5oz (100g) smoked
　　salmon
3½ tbsp (50ml) crème
　　fraîche
1 tsp black peppercorns
chopped chives, to
　　garnish
4 slices of whole wheat
　　toast, each spread
　　with 1 tsp butter

Lower the eggs into a pan of simmering water, making sure that the water covers them completely. Cook for 3½–5 minutes until soft-boiled. Drain and rinse under cold running water until they are cool enough to handle, then shell them.

While the eggs are cooking, chop the smoked salmon roughly and mix into the crème fraîche. Crack the black peppercorns using a pestle and mortar.

Halve the eggs and arrange on individual serving plates. Trickle the smoked salmon sauce over them. Scatter the cracked black peppercorns on top and garnish with chives. Serve at once with hot toast.

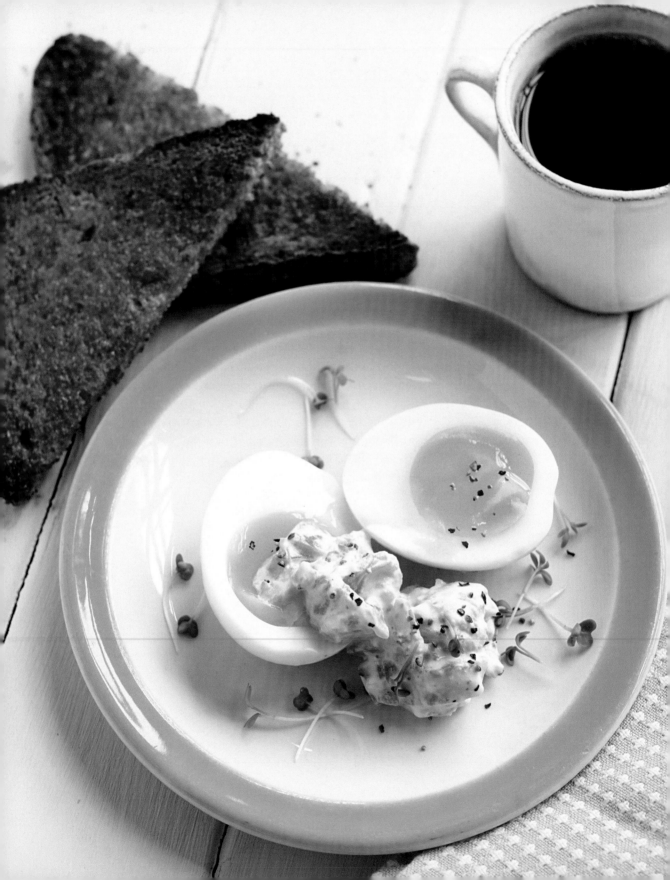

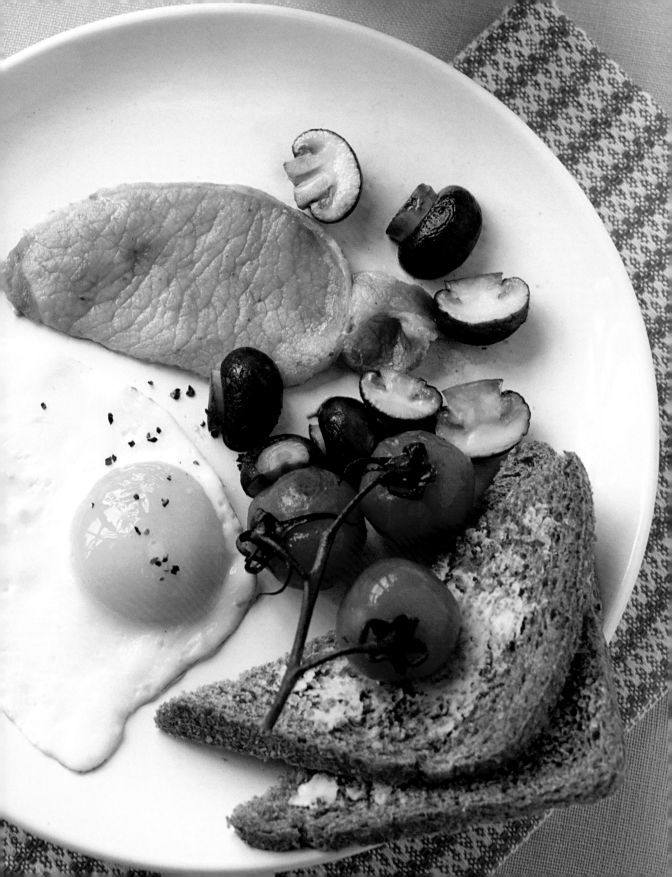

Low-Cal Eggs and Bacon

CALORIES PER SERVING: 276 with toast; 167 without toast

Serves 1 | Preparation time: 5 minutes | Cooking time: 10 minutes

Counting the calories doesn't mean you have to miss out on all the fun! With a few tweaks, you can enjoy all your favorites.

4 sprays low-cal
cooking spray
1 thin slice bacon,
trimmed of fat
4 cherry tomatoes,
halved
2 large cremini
mushrooms or
4 baby cremini
mushrooms,
quartered or halved
1 medium egg
salt and pepper
optional: 1 slice of whole
wheat toast, spread
with 1 tsp butter

Spray a large frying pan with the cooking spray and add the bacon, tomatoes and mushrooms. Cook over medium heat for 5 minutes, until softened. Season well with salt and pepper.

Spoon the mushrooms, tomatoes and bacon to the side and crack the egg into the middle of the pan. Cook over medium heat for a couple of minutes and then cover with a lid and continue to cook until the egg white is completely set. Check the seasoning and then serve with a slice of hot buttered toast, if desired.

Spiced Winter Fruit Compote

CALORIES PER SERVING: 290

Serves 2 | Preparation time: 10 minutes, plus cooling time | Cooking time: 50 minutes

Dried fruits are poached in apple juice and sumptuously scented with star anise and cinnamon. Served with thick Greek-style yogurt, this is an exotic way to begin your low-calorie day.

2oz (50g) dried pears
2oz (50g) dried figs
2oz (50g) dried
    apricots
2oz (50g) prunes
3.5oz (100ml) apple
    juice
1 star anise
½ cinnamon stick
optional: 2 tsp light
    muscovado sugar
3.75oz (110ml) Greek-
    style yogurt
a pinch of ground
    cinnamon

Put the fruit in a saucepan with the apple juice, star anise and cinnamon stick. Place over low heat and bring slowly to a boil.

Reduce the heat, cover the pan and simmer for 45 minutes until the fruits are plump and tender. Check the liquid during cooking to ensure there is a sufficient amount; add a little water if necessary.

Scrape the compote into a bowl. Taste for sweetness, and add a little sugar if necessary. Allow to cool to room temperature.

To serve, divide the compote between individual glass dishes. Top with yogurt and a light sprinkling of cinnamon.

Bircher Muesli

CALORIES PER SERVING: 317

Serves 1 | Preparation time: 5 minutes, plus resting time | Cooking time: 2 minutes

Deliciously moist oats with fresh apple and chopped dried figs rounded off with creamy yogurt. Make this the day before so the flavors have a chance to mingle.

3 tbsp rolled oats
1 dried fig, finely
    chopped
½ apple, grated
3oz (90ml) low-fat milk
2oz (50ml) low-fat plain
    yogurt
3 tsp slivered almonds
a pinch of ground
    cinnamon

Put the oats, chopped fig, apple, milk and yogurt in a bowl and mix together well. Chill in the fridge for a minimum of 30 minutes or overnight.

When ready to serve, toast the slivered almonds in a dry frying pan until just golden. Spoon the muesli into a bowl, top with the almonds and sprinkle with cinnamon.

Roasted Peaches with Pistachio Stuffing

CALORIES PER SERVING: 350

Serves 2 │ Preparation time: 15 minutes │ Cooking time: 20 minutes

Flavorful, fresh peaches are stuffed with a lightly spiced, crunchy filling of almond cookie crumbs and pale green pistachios, then baked until slightly soft. Choose peaches that are almost, but not quite, ripe enough to eat.

2oz (50g) almond
　　cookies
2.5oz (75g) shelled
　　pistachio nuts
1oz (25g) light
　　muscovado sugar
¼ tsp Chinese five spice
2 medium egg yolks
6 peaches
4 tbsp Greek-style
　　yogurt or crème
　　fraîche

Preheat the oven to 350˚F/180˚C. Roughly crush the almond cookies between two sheets of greaseproof paper, using a rolling pin or by processing briefly in a food processor. Finely chop the pistachios. Mix the crushed cookies and pistachios in a bowl with the sugar, spice and egg yolks.

Cut the peaches in half and remove the pits. Pile the nut filling into the peach halves and place them in a baking dish. Pour 5oz (150ml) water around the peaches and bake in the oven for 20 minutes or until the peaches are soft.

Transfer the stuffed peaches to individual serving plates and serve immediately, accompanied by the yogurt or crème fraîche.

Grilled Herrings with Oatmeal, Spinach and Almonds

CALORIES PER SERVING: 374

Serves 4 | Preparation time: 15 minutes | Cooking time: 15 minutes

Herrings are perfect for grilling, their oily, silvery skins turning beautifully crisp, charred and appetizing. These herrings have a moist spinach, almond and oatmeal stuffing, held together with a little melted cheddar.

4 herrings, boned
2 tsp balsamic or wine
    vinegar

for the stuffing
1½ tbsp (25g) butter
1 onion, peeled and
    finely chopped
1oz (25g) blanched
    almonds, chopped
4.5oz (125g) young
    spinach leaves,
    tough stalks
    removed
1oz (25g) medium
    oatmeal
2oz (50g) aged
    cheddar cheese,
    grated
salt and pepper
lemon wedges, to serve

To make the stuffing, melt the butter in a frying pan. Add the onion and almonds and fry for 3 minutes. Stir in the spinach and cook until just wilted.

Remove from the heat and stir in the oatmeal. Cool slightly, then add the cheese and a little seasoning.

Score the herrings, several times on each side. Sprinkle the vinegar inside the cavities and over the skins.

Spoon the prepared stuffing into the cavities and secure the opening with wooden cocktail sticks.

Preheat the grill to medium. Lightly oil a sheet of foil and use it to line a grill pan (this will stop the fish from sticking to the pan and also make it easier to clean up any filling that escapes during cooking). Place the herrings in the pan and grill for 15 minutes, turning over halfway through cooking.

Transfer the herrings to warmed serving plates and serve with lemon wedges.

Asparagus with Poached Eggs

CALORIES PER SERVING: 400

Serves 6 │ Preparation time: 20 minutes │ Cooking time: 40 minutes

The potatoes in this classic pairing make it a filling start to the day.

2lb (900g) asparagus

1¾lb (700g) small new
    potatoes, scrubbed

1⅓c (300ml crème
    fraîche or whipped
    heavy cream

3 tbsp tarragon vinegar

3 tbsp chopped
    tarragon, plus extra
    to garnish

6 medium eggs,
    refrigerated

salt and pepper

Peel the tough skin from the lower end of the asparagus stalks and then trim the stalks to an even length.

Fill a roasting pan with cold water and add a little salt. Bring to a boil and lay the asparagus in the pan. Boil for 10–15 minutes or longer, depending on the variety and thickness of the stalks.

Lift the asparagus out of the roasting pan and immediately plunge into a bowl of cold water to set the color and stop the cooking. Set aside.

Pour the asparagus water into a saucepan, add the potatoes and cook for 15–20 minutes until tender. Using a slotted spoon, transfer the potatoes to a colander and cool slightly. Reserve the water for poaching the eggs.

Mix the crème fraîche or whipped heavy cream with 1 tbsp of the vinegar. Stir in the tarragon, season, cover and refrigerate.

Slice the potatoes and arrange on serving plates. Season well. Drain and dry the asparagus on paper towels and lay over the potatoes.

Bring the reserved asparagus water to a rolling boil in a large shallow pan, adding the remaining 2 tbsp of vinegar and more water if necessary. Break the eggs into the bubbling water, then turn down to a bare simmer. Poach for 3–4 minutes— ideally they should still be quite soft. Lift out carefully, drain on paper towels and arrange on the asparagus. Season and serve at once with the tarragon cream and garnished with extra tarragon.

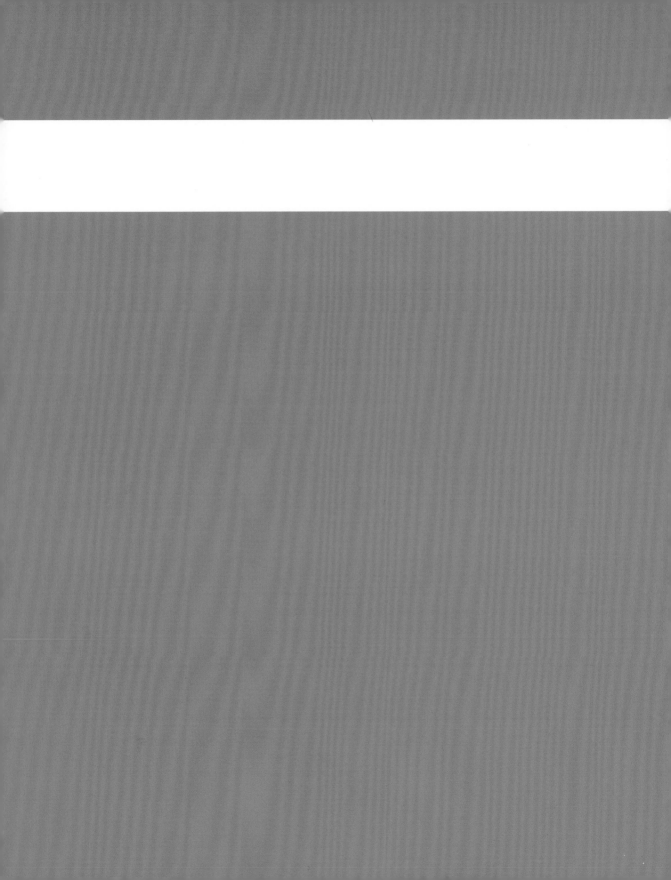

lunch

Mushroom Pâté with Madeira

CALORIES PER SERVING: 100

Serves 6 | Preparation time: 15 minutes, plus soaking time | Cooking time: 20–25 minutes

You can use any combination of mushrooms in this rich pâté, but try to include some flavorful wild ones or cultivated dark field mushrooms. Don't be tempted to use all button mushrooms, as the end result will lack color and flavor.

0.5oz (15g) dried porcini
    mushrooms
⅔c (150ml) warm
    low-fat milk
1 small onion
1 garlic clove
1½ tbsp (25g) butter
12oz (350g) mushrooms
½c (125g) ricotta
    cheese
1 tbsp Madeira
½ tsp balsamic vinegar
    or lemon juice
1 tsp Worcestershire
    sauce
freshly grated nutmeg,
    to taste
1–2 tbsp chopped
    flat-leaf parsley or
    cilantro, plus extra to
    garnish
coarse sea salt and
    pepper

Rinse the porcini under cold running water to wash away the grit, then place in a bowl. Pour on the warm milk and leave to soak for 20 minutes. Drain the porcini and chop finely.

Peel and finely chop the onion and garlic. Melt the butter in a saucepan, add the onion and garlic and fry gently for 5–10 minutes until softened and transparent.

Meanwhile, wipe the fresh mushrooms with a damp cloth to clean them, then chop finely.

Add the porcini and fresh mushrooms to the onion and garlic, increase the heat a little and cook, stirring occasionally, for about 15 minutes until the mushrooms are tender and reduced to a thick pulp. Leave to cool slightly.

Transfer the mushroom mixture to a food processor or bowl. Add the ricotta, Madeira, balsamic vinegar, Worcestershire sauce and nutmeg and process very briefly or stir until evenly mixed; the pâté should have a coarse texture. Stir in the chopped parsley or cilantro and adjust the seasoning.

Turn into a serving dish or individual ramekins and garnish with parsley or cilantro.

Spicy Grilled Eggplant Salad

CALORIES PER SERVING: 100

Serves 4 | Preparation time: 25 minutes, plus resting time | Cooking time: 10 minutes

For this unusual salad, baby eggplant slices are brushed with a sweet soy glaze, then grilled until charred and tender and tossed with green beans in a sesame and lime dressing. Serve the salad while it is still warm.

4 baby eggplants
2 tsp sea salt
2 tbsp soy sauce
2 tsp Thai fish sauce
1 tsp hot chili sauce
1 tsp lemon juice
½ tsp ground cumin
½ tsp honey
4.5oz (125g) green
    beans

for the dressing
1 tbsp peanut or
    sunflower oil
1 tsp sesame oil
1 tbsp lime juice
a pinch of sugar

to serve
½ lettuce
2 tbsp lime juice
sesame seeds
mint leaves

Trim the eggplants and cut each one into 4 slices. Place the eggplants in a colander set over a plate and sprinkle over the salt. Leave for 30 minutes so the eggplants can release their bitter juices.

Meanwhile, in a small bowl mix together the sweet soy sauce, fish sauce, chili sauce, lemon juice, cumin and honey. Set aside.

Trim the beans and cut into 2in (5cm) lengths. Bring a large pan of lightly salted water to a rolling boil, plunge in the green beans, return to the boil and cook for 3 minutes until the beans are tender. Immediately drain and refresh the beans under cold running water. Drain again.

Preheat the grill to high. Rinse the eggplants to remove the salt and pat dry. Place on a rack over the grill pan and brush with half the soy sauce mixture. Grill as close to the heat as possible for 2–3 minutes. Turn the slices over, brush with the remaining soy mixture and grill until charred and tender.

Whisk the ingredients for the dressing together until evenly blended. Toss the green beans with half of the dressing.

Tear the lettuce into bite-size pieces, toss with the lime juice and arrange on individual serving plates. Top with the eggplant slices and beans, then drizzle the remaining dressing on top. Scatter some sesame seeds and mint leaves on top as well and serve at once.

Sugar Snap Peas with a Minted Lemon Dip

CALORIES PER SERVING: 105

Serves 4 | Preparation time: 10 minutes | Cooking time: 5–10 minutes

Sugar snap peas are available all year round. In this low-calorie lunch they are served with a light crème fraîche dipping sauce, flavored with fresh mint and lemon.

1lb (450g) sugar snap
    peas

for the sauce
4 tbsp crème fraîche
1 tbsp finely shredded
    or chopped mint
finely grated zest and
    juice of
    ½ lemon
3oz (90ml) Greek-style
    yogurt
coarse sea salt and
    pepper

Trim the sugar snap peas, then steam or cook them in boiling water until just tender.

Prepare the sauce: put all the ingredients in a bowl, reserving a little lemon zest to garnish. Stir together and season with salt and pepper, to taste.

Drain the sugar snap peas and spoon the yogurt sauce into a small serving dish. Garnish with the reserved lemon zest and serve at once.

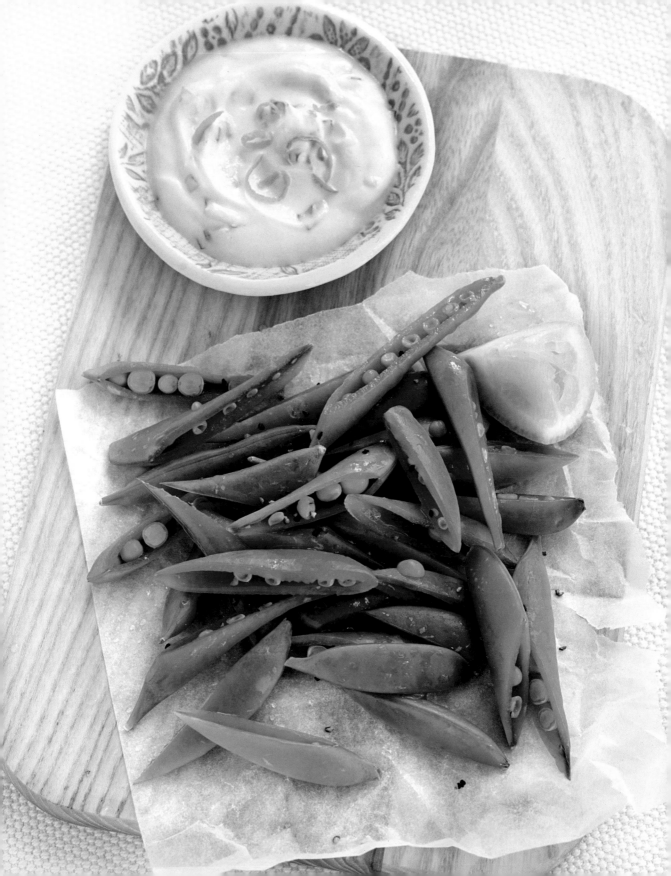

Spicy Beef Soup

CALORIES PER SERVING: 115

Serves 4 | Preparation time: 30 minutes | Cooking time: 15 minutes

A comforting and surprisingly filling soup with lots of flavor—add a few chili flakes for even more heat. Make sure you use lean pieces of beef; cube steak is perfect for this dish.

5c (1.2 liters) vegetable
    stock
1 red chile, deseeded
    and diced
1 tbsp Thai fish sauce
2 tbsp rice vinegar
1 tbsp chili sauce
3.5oz (100g) baby
    cremini mushrooms,
    finely sliced
1 red pepper, finely
    sliced
3.5oz (100g) baby corn,
    finely sliced
1 small carrot, finely
    sliced
7oz (200g) lean beef,
    cut into strips
1 tsp chili oil
2 tbsp cilantro leaves

Put the vegetable stock into a pan and add the chile, fish sauce, vinegar and chili sauce. Bring to a boil and simmer gently for 10 minutes.

Add the mushrooms, pepper, corn and carrot, and simmer for another 10 minutes.

Stir in the beef strips and continue to simmer, until cooked to your liking. Ladle into four bowls and serve with a dash of chili oil and the cilantro leaves.

Grilled Jumbo Prawns with Chili Soy Sauce

CALORIES PER SERVING: 120

Serves 4 | Preparation time: 20 minutes, plus marinating | Cooking time: 20 minutes

This is a dish that definitely requires a napkin! It's a messy business, but what could be better than dipping succulent grilled prawns into a rich, tangy dip?

12 large raw jumbo
    prawns, peeled and
    deveined
1 tbsp chopped cilantro
lime wedges, to serve

for the marinade
1 garlic clove, peeled
1 red chile, deseeded
1 tbsp sesame oil
2 tbsp dark soy sauce
grated zest and juice of
    2 limes
1 tbsp soft brown sugar

for the chili soy sauce
1 tsp crushed chili flakes
1 tbsp lime juice
2 tbsp dark soy sauce
1 tbsp Thai fish sauce
2 tbsp soft brown sugar

To prepare the prawns, use a sharp knife to slit each one down the back and remove the black intestinal vein. Rinse in cold water and dry on paper towels, then place in a shallow non-reactive dish. To make the marinade, finely chop the garlic and chile and mix with the remaining ingredients. Pour over the prawns and stir well to coat. Cover the dish and leave to marinate in a cool place for at least 4 hours, preferably overnight.

For the chili soy sauce, place all the ingredients in a small pan with 2 tablespoons of cold water and bring to a boil, stirring until the sugar is dissolved. Remove the pan from the heat and leave to cool.

Just before serving, preheat the grill to medium. Transfer the prawns to the grill pan and grill as close to the heat as possible for 6–8 minutes, turning and basting frequently with the marinade juices, until the prawns are pink and lightly charred.

Transfer the prawns to a warmed serving platter and scatter the chopped cilantro on top. Serve with lime wedges and the chili sauce for dipping.

Tuscan Bean Soup with Toasted Garlic

CALORIES PER SERVING: 159

Serves 6 | Preparation time: 20 minutes, plus soaking time | Cooking time: 1 hour 10 minutes

A substantial white bean soup. If the soup is thicker than you like, thin it down with a little extra water or stock. This makes a lot of soup, but it's excellent to freeze—reheat it straight from frozen.

8oz (225g) dried white haricot or cannellini beans
4 garlic cloves, peeled
2 tbsp (50ml) olive oil
1–2 tbsp chopped flat-leaf parsley
salt and pepper

Put the dried beans in a bowl and pour on enough cold water to cover. Leave to soak overnight.

The next day, preheat the oven to 325°F/170°C. Drain the beans and place in a flameproof casserole. Cover with cold water to 2in (5cm) above the beans. Bring to a boil, then cover tightly and bake in the oven for about 1 hour or until tender (see note). Keep them in their cooking liquid.

Meanwhile, finely chop half the garlic and thinly slice the remainder.

Transfer half of the beans and liquid to a food processor or blender and process until smooth. Add this purée to the beans in the casserole and stir well.

Heat half the olive oil in a frying pan, add the chopped garlic and fry gently until soft and golden. Stir into the soup and reheat until boiling. Simmer gently for 10 minutes. Taste and season well with salt and pepper. Pour into a warmed tureen or individual soup bowls.

Heat the remaining olive oil in the frying pan and fry the sliced garlic until golden. Spoon over the soup and serve at once, sprinkled with the chopped parsley.

Note: The cooking time depends on the freshness of the beans. Older beans will take longer to cook. Begin testing them after 45 minutes.

Chilled Beet and Apple Soup

CALORIES PER SERVING: 160

Serves 4 | Preparation time: 10 minutes

A cool, deep crimson soup that's as wonderfully refreshing to eat as it looks. Serve it topped with a dollop of the minted cucumber cream.

12oz (350g) cooked, peeled beets

juice of ½ lemon

2½c (600ml) unsweetened apple juice, chilled

7oz (200g) Greek-style yogurt, chilled

cayenne pepper, to taste

4in (10cm) piece cucumber

6 mint leaves, finely chopped

salt and pepper

8 chives, to garnish

Slice the beets and place in a food processor or blender. Add the lemon juice, half the apple juice and half the yogurt. Process for a couple of minutes until smooth.

Pour the beet mixture into a mixing bowl, stir in the rest of the apple juice and season to taste with salt, pepper and cayenne pepper. Chill until you are ready to serve, then pour into individual bowls.

To make the cucumber cream, grate the cucumber and stir into the remaining yogurt. Stir the mint into the mixture. Spoon some cucumber cream into the middle of each serving and sprinkle with a little cayenne pepper. Snip the chives over the top to garnish.

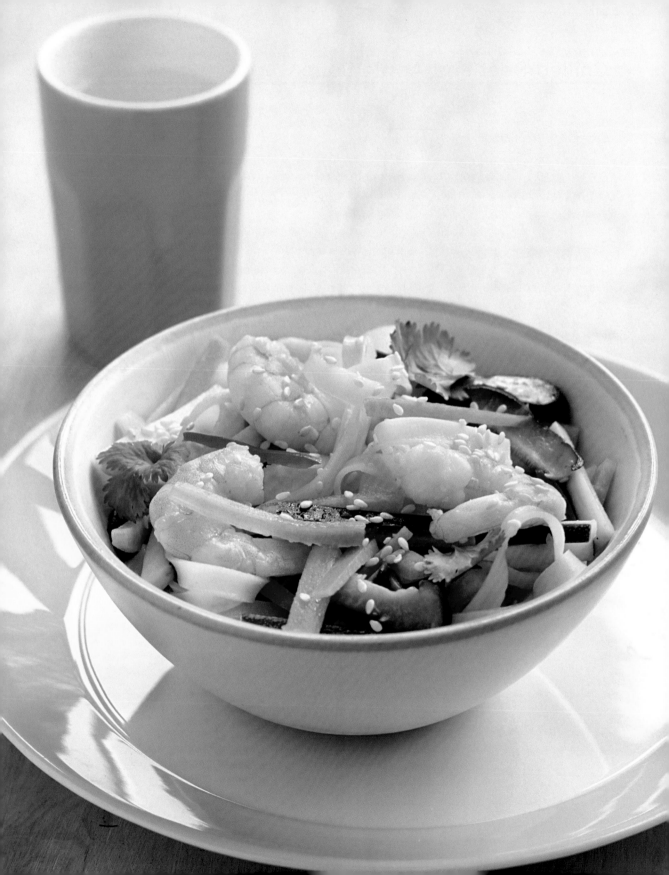

Prawn and Rice Noodle Salad

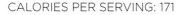

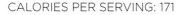

CALORIES PER SERVING: 171

Serves 4 │ Preparation time: 15 minutes │ Cooking time: 1 minute

This is a very pretty Thai-style salad, packed with flavor. The dressing is deliciously sharp and sweet and the rice noodles are pleasingly low in calories.

2oz (50g) dried rice
    noodles
2.5oz (75g) shiitake
    mushrooms
1 large carrot
1 large zucchini
6.2oz (175g) large
    cooked prawns,
    peeled
1 tbsp toasted sesame
    seeds
2 tbsp chopped cilantro

for the dressing
2 garlic cloves
1 tbsp light soy sauce
2 tbsp sugar
1 tbsp wine vinegar
1 tbsp sesame oil
1 red chile

First make the dressing. Crush the garlic and mix with the soy sauce, sugar, wine vinegar and sesame oil in a small bowl. Cut the chile in half lengthwise, remove the seeds, then cut into very fine strips. Mix into the dressing.

Cut the noodles into 10cm lengths. Cook in boiling water according to the packet instructions. Drain thoroughly and refresh under cold running water. Drain again.

Trim the mushrooms and slice finely. Add to the dressing and mix thoroughly.

Cut the carrot and zucchini into fine julienne or matchstick strips.

Place the noodles in a bowl and add the mushrooms with the dressing, the carrot and zucchini, and the prawns. Toss the salad well to combine all the ingredients. Sprinkle with the sesame seeds and chopped cilantro to serve.

Chickpeas with Ginger and Tomato

CALORIES PER SERVING: 175

Serves 6 | Preparation time: 5 minutes, plus overnight soaking | Cooking time: 2 hours

The flavor in this dish is improved if it is made the day before required and reheated. If you don't have the time for soaking and cooking dried chickpeas, use canned ones instead—they work equally well (see note).

8oz (225g) dried
   chickpeas
2in (5cm) piece fresh
   ginger root
2 garlic cloves
1 tbsp olive oil
2 tsp garam masala
1 x 15oz (400g) can of
   chopped tomatoes
2 spring onions
5oz (150ml) Greek-style
   yogurt
1 tsp mild curry paste
2 tbsp chopped mint
2 tbsp chopped cilantro
salt and pepper
cilantro and mint sprigs,
   to garnish

Put the chickpeas in a large bowl and pour on enough cold water to cover. Leave to soak overnight.

The next day, drain the chickpeas and put them in a large saucepan with enough fresh cold water to cover. Bring to a boil and boil steadily for 10 minutes, then lower the heat and simmer for about 1½ hours, until the chickpeas are really tender, adding salt toward the end of the cooking time. Drain thoroughly.

Peel and finely chop the ginger and garlic. Heat the oil in the saucepan and add the ginger, garlic and garam masala. Sauté for 2 minutes, then add the tomatoes and chickpeas and bring to a boil. Reduce the heat and simmer gently for 15 minutes.

Meanwhile, trim and finely chop the spring onions. Place in a bowl with the yogurt, curry paste, mint and cilantro. Mix thoroughly and season liberally with salt and pepper.

Turn the chickpeas into a serving bowl and swirl in the yogurt mixture. Serve immediately, garnished with cilantro and mint sprigs.

Note: Replace the dried chickpeas with two 14oz (400g) cans of chickpeas. Drain and rinse thoroughly under cold running water and add with the tomatoes as above.

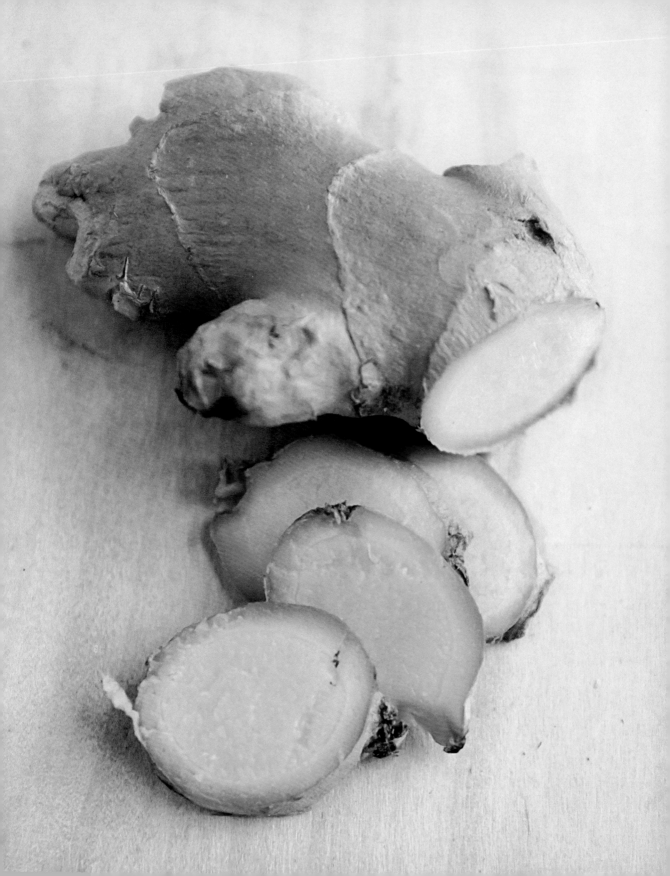

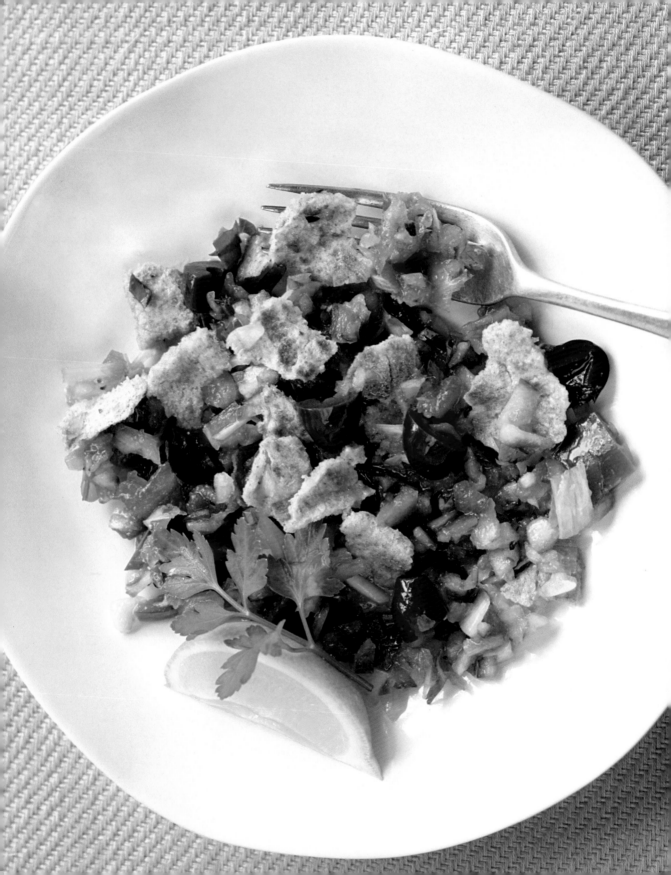

Fattoush

CALORIES PER SERVING: 180

Serves 4 │ Preparation time: 15 minutes │ Cooking time: 3 minutes

A gloriously flavorful Middle Eastern salad that's reminiscent of a solid gazpacho. This makes a wonderfully filling lunch and is easy to transport in a lunchbox.

4 tomatoes
½ cucumber
4 spring onions
1 small green pepper
1 garlic clove, crushed
juice of ½ lemon
2 tbsp finely chopped
    flat-leaf parsley
2 tbsp roughly torn
    mint leaves
3 tbsp olive oil
1 whole wheat pita
    bread
12 black olives, pitted
    and chopped
salt and pepper

Preheat the grill to medium. Put the tomatoes into a heatproof bowl and pour on boiling water to cover. Leave for 1 minute, then drain and remove the skins. Cut them up roughly and place in a food processor or blender. Cut the cucumber roughly and place in the food processor too.

Trim and roughly chop the spring onions. Halve, core and deseed the green pepper, then roughly chop the flesh. Add the spring onions and green pepper to the food processor with the garlic and lemon juice. Process to a chunky purée.

Turn the mixture into a bowl and stir in the chopped parsley, mint, olive oil, and salt and pepper to taste.

Toast the pita bread briefly on both sides. Break into small pieces and scatter over the salad.

Transfer the salad to a serving dish and sprinkle with black olives.

Note: You can make this salad by hand if you prefer, chopping all the vegetables finely, but it will take a little longer.

Fennel and Orange Salad

CALORIES PER SERVING: 185

Serves 4 | Preparation time: 15 minutes

Fennel with orange is a fairly classic combination, though here it is enhanced with a rich olive pesto, which works particularly well with the orange. Blood oranges are the ideal choice when in season, as they have a delicious, sweet flavor and pretty ruby-colored flesh.

2 large oranges
1 medium fennel bulb
1 small red onion
2oz (50g) arugula
    leaves

for the dressing
0.5oz (15g) pitted black
    olives
1 sun-dried tomato in
    oil, drained
1 small garlic clove,
    crushed
½ tbsp chopped flat-
    leaf parsley
4 tbsp extra virgin olive oil
2 tsp balsamic vinegar
salt and pepper

First make the dressing. Roughly chop the olives and sun-dried tomato. Place in a blender or food processor with the garlic, parsley and 1 tablespoon of oil. Blend to form a fairly smooth paste. Transfer to a bowl and whisk in the remaining oil, vinegar and seasoning to taste.

Peel the oranges, removing all the white pith, then cut into segments between the membranes and place in a large bowl.

Discard the tough outer layer from the fennel, then slice very thinly. Finely slice the onion.

Add the fennel, onion and arugula to the oranges. Pour the dressing on top and toss well until evenly coated. Serve at once.

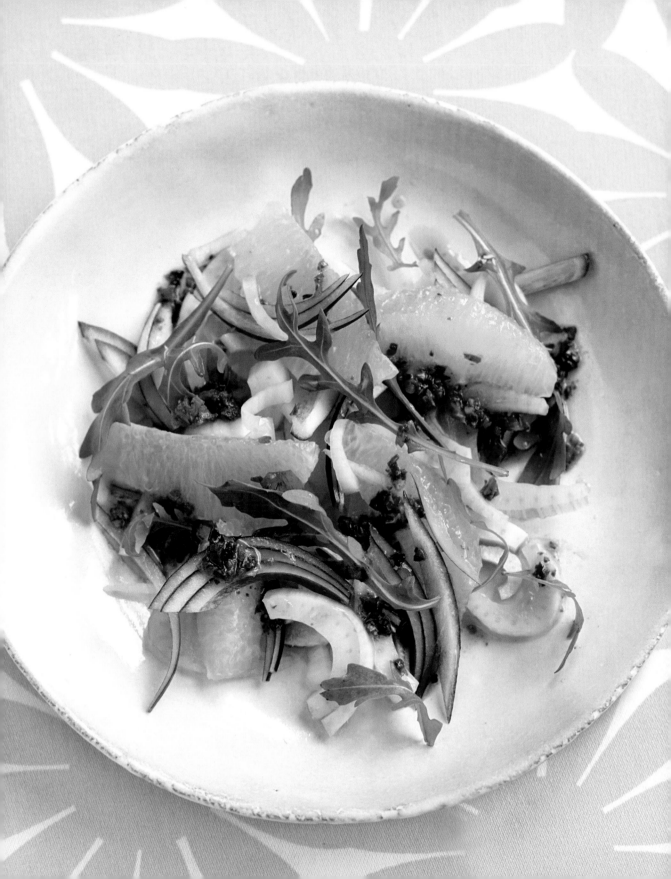

Spicy Parsnip and Carrot Soup with Cumin

CALORIES PER SERVING: 200

Serves 4 | Preparation time: 15 minutes | Cooking time: 15–20 minutes

A warming vegetarian soup, with a delicious hint of spicy cumin seeds. As the parsnip and carrot purée is sufficient to thicken the soup, there are no added calories in the form of flour. For optimum flavor, use homemade vegetable stock.

1lb (450g) parsnips
8oz (225g) carrots
2 tbsp olive oil
1 onion, peeled and
    finely chopped
1 tbsp curry powder
1½c (350ml) vegetable
    stock
10oz (300ml) low-fat
    milk
salt and pepper
2 tsp cumin seeds,
    to garnish

Peel the parsnips, cut in half and remove the woody stems. Peel the carrots. Cut the parsnips and carrots into even-sized pieces.

Heat the oil in a heavy-based saucepan, add the vegetables, including the onion, and stir to lightly coat in the oil. Cover and cook for a few minutes until the vegetables are slightly softened. Sprinkle in the curry powder and cook, stirring, for 1 minute.

Stir in the vegetable stock and milk, and season with salt and pepper. Bring to a boil, then reduce the heat to a gentle simmer and cook for 15–20 minutes until the vegetables are soft.

Allow the soup to cool a little, then transfer to a blender or food processor and work until smooth. If the consistency is a little too thick for your liking, add a splash of vegetable stock.

Toast the cumin seeds by gently frying them in a non-stick pan, or spread on a baking sheet and broil under a medium heat. Meanwhile, return the soup to the saucepan and reheat gently. Serve the soup in warmed bowls, garnished with a sprinkling of cumin seeds.

Green Bean and Omelet Ribbon Salad

CALORIES PER SERVING: 210

Serves 4 | Preparation time: 15 minutes | Cooking time: 10 minutes

Thin strips of omelet festoon slim green beans in this pretty salad, which is enhanced by a vigorous dressing full of Mediterranean flavors.

2 medium eggs
3 tbsp (50ml) olive oil
12oz (350g) green
    beans
1 large garlic clove
1 tsp red wine vinegar
1 tsp balsamic vinegar
2 sun-dried tomatoes,
    in oil, drained
1 tsp capers
salt and pepper

Break the eggs into a bowl, season with salt and pepper and beat lightly with a fork. Smear a 7–8in (18–20cm) frying pan (preferably non-stick) with a little olive oil and place over medium heat. When it is hot, pour in half the egg mixture and swirl the pan to spread the mixture quickly. It will set almost immediately into a thin omelet. Turn out on to a plate and repeat with the remaining egg, turning it out on to a separate plate.

Trim the green beans and cook them in a little boiling salted water for about 5 minutes. Drain and spread in a serving dish.

Peel the garlic and slice very thinly. Heat 1 tbsp of the oil in a pan, add the garlic and fry very briefly until it sizzles—be careful not to let it brown too much as it will make the dish taste bitter. Immediately add the remaining oil and vinegars to stop the cooking and swirl vigorously together.

Chop the sun-dried tomatoes; chop the capers coarsely. Swirl them into the dressing and season with pepper, adding a little salt only if needed. Pour the dressing over the salad.

Slice the omelets into ¼in (0.5cm) ribbons and curl them loosely over the beans.

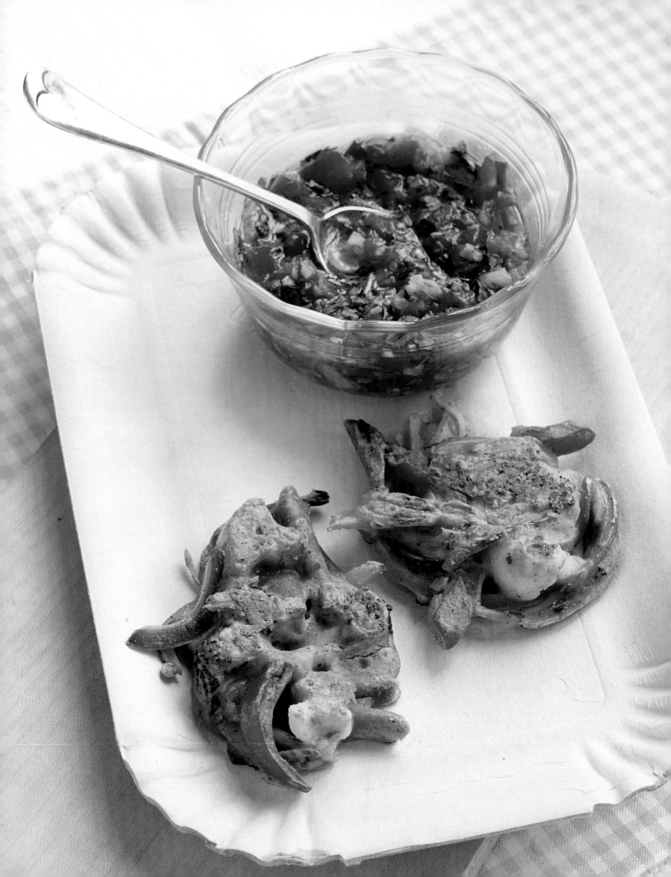

Indian Spiced Fritters with Cilantro Chutney

CALORIES PER SERVING: 215 (20 calories per fritter)

Serves 2 │ Preparation time: 30 minutes, plus resting time │ Cooking time: 10–20 minutes

Gently spiced veggies with a fresh chutney dip, this is irresistible Indian-style finger food.

10oz (275g) vegetables, such as onion, cauliflower, carrots, green beans, red pepper
1 tsp cumin seeds
1 tsp cilantro seeds
½ tsp chili flakes
2.5oz (75g) chickpea flour
1 tsp garam masala
½ tsp salt
1 tbsp vegetable oil

for the cilantro chutney
1 shallot, peeled
1 small garlic clove, peeled
1 hot red chile
½ tsp salt
1 tbsp lime or lemon juice
2.25oz (65g) roasted red pepper in oil, drained
2 tbsp chopped cilantro

Prepare the vegetables: peel and roughly chop the onion; divide the cauliflower into small florets and halve; roughly chop the carrots and green beans; cut the red pepper into bite-size pieces. Blanch in a pan of boiling water, until tender but with a slight bite.

Crush the cumin, cilantro seeds and chili flakes, using a pestle and mortar. Heat a frying pan, add the spices and toast for 2 minutes, stirring.

Mix the chickpea flour, garam masala and salt in a bowl. Add the spice mixture, then gradually stir in about ⅓ to ½c (75–100ml) cold water, or enough to make a thick batter. Beat vigorously with a wooden spoon or a balloon whisk to remove any lumps. Leave the batter to stand for about 30 minutes.

Meanwhile, make the chutney. Quarter the shallot and place in a food processor or blender with all of the other ingredients, except the red pepper and cilantro. Process until well mixed but still retaining some texture, then transfer to a bowl. Coarsely chop the red pepper and stir into the chutney along with the cilantro. Cover and leave to stand for 30 minutes to let the flavors develop.

Heat the oil in a non-stick frying pan. Stir the vegetables into the batter. Place small spoonfuls of the battered vegetables in the frying pan and fry until golden underneath. Flip over and fry on the other side until golden and cooked through. Drain on paper towels and keep warm. Continue to cook until all the batter is used up, adding more oil to the pan as you need to—you should make about 20. Serve the spicy fritters piping hot with the cilantro chutney.

Asian-Style Chicken Noodle Soup

CALORIES PER SERVING: 229

Serves 2 | Preparation time: 15 minutes | Cooking time: 35 minutes

There's nothing more soothing and comforting than a steaming bowl of chicken noodle soup. Add more chile if you like it fiery.

1 skinless chicken thigh,
    on the bone
1 lemongrass stalk,
    finely sliced
1in (2.5cm) piece fresh
    ginger root, cut into
    slivers
1 red chile, sliced
1 garlic clove, sliced
2oz (50g) egg noodles
1 carrot, cut into sticks
3 stems purple
    sprouting broccoli or
    broccolini, roughly
    chopped
¼ red pepper, cut into
    strips
2oz (50g) bean sprouts
1 tbsp miso paste
1 tsp sesame oil
1 spring onion, finely
    sliced, to garnish

Put the chicken, lemongrass, ginger, chile and garlic in a pan with 600ml water. Cover and bring to a boil. Turn the heat down to low and simmer for 20 minutes.

Lift the chicken out of the pan and put on a cutting board. Strain the stock into another pan, discard the aromatics, and add 1¼c (300ml) water. Shred the chicken.

Bring the stock up to a boil and add the noodles, carrot and broccoli or broccolini. Simmer for 3 minutes.

Return the chicken to the pan and add the pepper and bean sprouts and stir in the miso paste. Simmer for another minute until the chicken is heated through and the vegetables are just tender.

Ladle between two bowls, stir in the sesame oil and sprinkle with the spring onion.

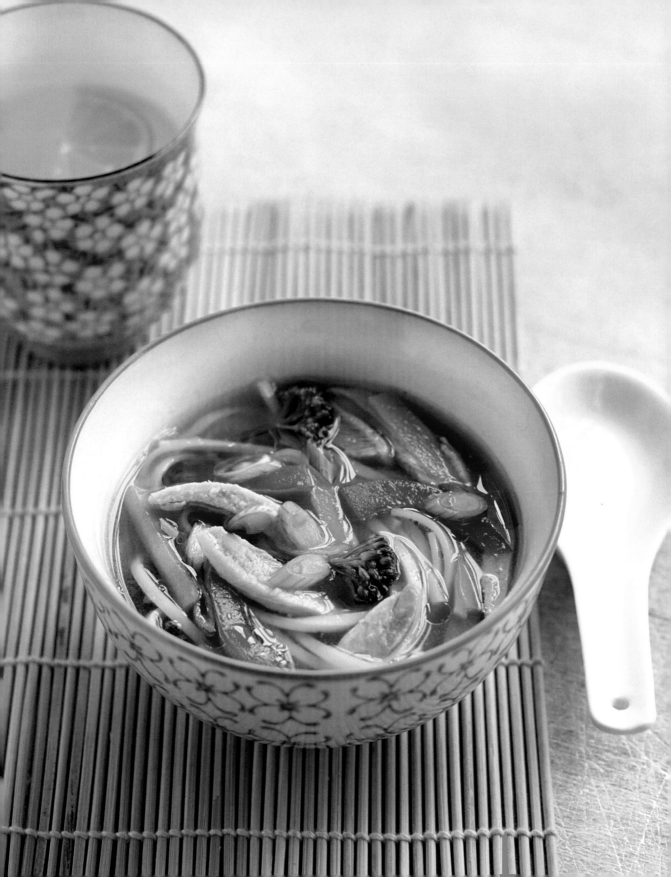

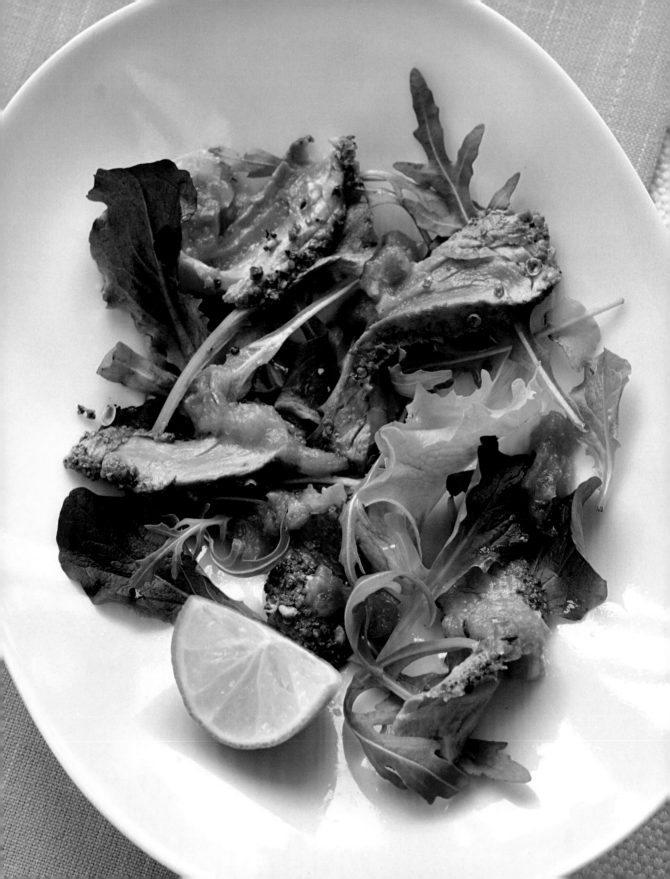

Beef Salad with a Sweet and Sour Dressing

CALORIES PER SERVING: 230

Serves 4 | Preparation time: 35 minutes, plus marinating time | Cooking time: 30–35 minutes

This recipe is based on a Thai dish called *larp*, which is similar to beef tartare. Here the beef is seared as a whole fillet, then sliced and served on a bed of tangy salad greens.

8oz (225g) fillet steak
1 tbsp Szechuan
    peppercorns
1 tsp ground black
    pepper
1 tsp ground cilantro
¼ tsp Chinese five spice
4.5oz (125g) salad greens
1 tbsp sesame seeds
lime wedges, to serve

for the dressing
8oz (225g) shallots,
    peeled
4 garlic cloves, peeled
2 large chiles, deseeded
1in (2.5cm) piece fresh
    ginger root, peeled
1 lemongrass stalk
1 tsp cumin seeds
3 tbsp sunflower oil
1 tbsp tamarind paste
1 tbsp light soy sauce or
    Thai fish sauce
2 tsp sugar

Preheat the oven to 400°F/200°C. Wash and dry the beef. Roughly grind the Szechuan peppercorns, using a pestle and mortar or spice grinder, and mix with the black pepper, ground cilantro and five spice. Spread on a cutting board. Press the steak down into the spice mixture, turning to coat well on both sides. Cover and leave to marinate in the fridge for 2 hours.

Meanwhile, prepare the dressing. Halve any large shallots; roughly chop the garlic, chiles and ginger; finely chop the lemongrass. Place these ingredients in a small roasting pan with the cumin seeds. Pour over the oil and toss well until evenly combined. Transfer to the oven and roast for 30 minutes until browned and softened. Allow to cool slightly.

Transfer the roasted aromatics to a food processor and add the tamarind paste, soy or fish sauce and the sugar. Purée to form a rough paste, adding a little water if it seems too thick. Taste and add a little salt if necessary.

Brush a griddle or heavy-based frying pan with a little oil and heat. As soon as the oil starts to smoke, add the beef fillet and sear by pressing down hard with a spatula. Fry for 1 minute, turn the steak and repeat on the second side. Remove from the pan and leave to rest for 2 minutes.

Divide the salad greens among individual serving plates. Thinly slice the beef fillet and arrange on the plates. Spoon on a little of the dressing and scatter the sesame seeds on top. Serve at once, with lime wedges.

Baked Fennel with Lemon and Olives

CALORIES PER SERVING: 230

Serves 4 | Preparation time: 15 minutes | Cooking time: 45 minutes

Fennel bulbs are braised to tender sweetness with smoky black olives and lemon juice.
This dish is equally delicious served hot or cold.

3 large fennel bulbs, or
    4 medium
grated zest and juice of
    1 lemon
6 tbsp olive oil
20 black or green olives
salt and pepper
2 tbsp chopped flat-leaf
    parsley, to garnish

Preheat the oven to 400°F/200°C. Trim the fennel and cut away any bruised parts. Cut off the fibrous tops, halve the bulbs lengthways and cut out the core. Cut larger bulbs into quarters.

Place the fennel halves or quarters cut-side up in a baking dish. Mix the lemon zest and juice with the olive oil, salt and pepper.

Pour the lemon mixture over the fennel, scatter over the olives and bake in the oven for 15 minutes. Turn the fennel and bake for another 15 minutes. Turn once more and bake for a final 15 minutes until tender. Serve sprinkled with the parsley.

Note: For a softer texture, blanch the fennel quarters in boiling water for 2 minutes and drain well before baking.

Mushroom and Artichoke Soup with Walnuts

CALORIES PER SERVING: 250

Serves 4 | Preparation time: 20 minutes, plus soaking time | Cooking time: 1½ hours

Jerusalem artichokes have a very distinctive flavor. The intense mushroom stock combines beautifully with the artichokes, and the walnuts add texture to the finished soup. This soup is great to freeze and can be cooked straight from frozen.

0.5oz (15g) dried porcini mushrooms

5oz (150ml) boiling water

1½ tbsp (25g) butter

1 tbsp chopped fresh thyme leaves

1 small onion, chopped

1lb (450g) cremini mushrooms, chopped

3oz (90ml) dry sherry

5c (1.2 liters) vegetable stock

1lb (450g) Jerusalem artichokes

1 garlic clove

2 tbsp walnut oil, plus extra to drizzle

1oz (25g) walnuts, chopped and toasted

salt and pepper

thyme sprigs, to garnish

Put the dried porcinis into a bowl, pour over the boiling water and let soak for 30 minutes. Drain, reserving the liquid.

Melt the butter in a saucepan, add the thyme and onion and fry gently for 10 minutes until soft but not browned. Increase the heat, add the cremini mushrooms and porcinis and stir-fry for 2 minutes. Add the sherry and boil rapidly until well reduced.

Add the vegetable stock and reserved porcini stock and bring to a boil. Cover and simmer gently for 20 minutes until the stock is rich tasting and the mushrooms have lost all their flavor.

Meanwhile, scrub the artichokes and cut away the knobby bits. Peel, then dice the flesh. Chop the garlic. Heat the oil in a large pan, add the artichokes and garlic and fry for 10 minutes, stirring, until evenly browned.

Strain the mushroom liquid through a fine sieve and add to the artichokes. Bring to a boil, cover and simmer for 35–40 minutes until the artichokes are cooked. Transfer to a blender or food processor and purée until very smooth.

Return the soup to the pan and heat gently for 5 minutes. Season with salt and pepper, to taste, and spoon into warmed soup bowls. Scatter the toasted nuts over the soup and drizzle with walnut oil. Serve at once, garnished with thyme.

Arugula and Goat Cheese
with Roasted Pepper Salsa

CALORIES PER SERVING: 255

Serves 4 | Preparation time: 20 minutes | Cooking time: 25 minutes

Here a delicious, juicy pepper salsa serves as the perfect partner for goat cheese.
Roasting the peppers first not only sweetens them but also ensures that their skin
falls away from the flesh, making them far easier to peel.

1 small red pepper
1 small orange pepper
3 tbsp extra virgin
    olive oil
1 small red onion
1 garlic clove
2 ripe plum tomatoes
1½ tbsp balsamic
    vinegar
a pinch of sugar
2 tbsp chopped fresh
    chervil
4.5oz (125g) goat
    cheese
4.5oz (125g) arugula
    leaves
2 tbsp pine nuts,
    toasted
salt and pepper

Preheat the oven to 450°F/230°C. Brush the peppers with
a little oil and place in a roasting pan. Roast in the oven for
20 minutes, turning once, until charred. Transfer to a bowl,
cover with a towel and set aside until cool enough to handle.

Carefully peel the peppers over the bowl to catch the
juices, then discard the seeds. Dice the pepper flesh and
add to the juices.

Finely chop the onion and garlic. Immerse the tomatoes in
boiling water for 30 seconds, then remove and peel away
the skins. Halve, deseed and dice the tomato flesh.

Heat 1 tablespoon of the oil in a small pan, add the onion
and garlic, and fry for about 3 minutes until softened. Add
the diced tomatoes and fry gently for another 2 minutes.
Add to the peppers, toss to mix and set aside to cool.

Combine the remaining oil with the vinegar, sugar, chervil and
seasoning. Pour over the pepper mixture and toss to mix.

Thinly slice the goat cheese. Divide the arugula among
individual serving plates and arrange the cheese in the
center. Spoon some of the salsa over the cheese and drizzle
the rest liberally over the arugula. Scatter the pine nuts on
top and serve at once.

Curried Carrot and Split Pea Soup

CALORIES PER SERVING: 260

Serves 4 | Preparation time: 35 minutes, plus soaking time | Cooking time: 1–1¼ hours

There is undoubtedly something warming about a curried lentil or split pea soup. A tangy cilantro and lime butter complements this soup perfectly, giving it a delicious finish. Alternatively you could omit the flavored butter and simply sprinkle the soup with chopped cilantro instead.

2oz (50g) yellow split peas, soaked overnight in cold water
1 tbsp sunflower oil
1 small onion, chopped
1 garlic clove, chopped
1 red chile, deseeded and chopped
1 tsp grated fresh ginger root
1½ tsp hot curry paste
8oz (225g) carrots, peeled and chopped
1 potato, peeled and chopped
salt and pepper

for the cilantro and lime butter
3½ tbsp (50g) butter, softened
grated zest and juice of 1 lime
1½ tsp chopped cilantro

Drain the split peas, rinse well and place in a large saucepan with 6⅓c (1.5 liters) of cold water. Bring to a boil and boil steadily for 10 minutes. Reduce the heat, cover and simmer gently for 30 minutes.

Meanwhile, make the cilantro and lime butter. In a bowl, beat the butter with the lime zest and juice, cilantro and a little pepper, until evenly combined. Form into a log shape on a piece of parchment paper, wrap in foil and chill in the fridge until required.

Heat the oil in a pan, add the onion, garlic, chile and ginger and fry, stirring frequently, for 10 minutes until evenly browned. Stir in the curry paste, carrots and potato and fry for another 5 minutes.

Add the curried vegetable mixture to the split peas. Return to a boil, cover and simmer for another 35 minutes until the vegetables and peas are tender. Transfer to a blender or food processor and purée until fairly smooth. Return to the pan, season with salt and pepper, to taste, and heat through.

Unwrap the butter and cut into thin slices. Pour the soup into warmed serving bowls and serve each portion topped with two slices of the flavored butter.

Vegetable Couscous

CALORIES PER SERVING: 260

Serves 4 │ Preparation time: 15 minutes │ Cooking time: 15 minutes

For this quick Moroccan-style dish, couscous grains are steamed over a nourishing spicy vegetable stew. Use quick-cook couscous—which needs to be moistened before cooking but doesn't require lengthy soaking—and vary the vegetables as you like.

8oz (225g) quick-cook
    couscous
8oz (225g) eggplant
6oz (175g) zucchinis
6oz (175g) carrots,
    peeled
1 large onion
1 tbsp oil
2 garlic cloves, crushed
2 tsp ground cumin
½ tsp mild chili
    seasoning
½ tsp ground ginger
4 tbsp tomato purée
1 bay leaf
7 oz (200g) canned
    chickpeas
3c (750ml) vegetable
    stock
salt and pepper
chopped flat-leaf
    parsley, to garnish

Moisten the couscous according to the packet instructions. Cut the eggplant and zucchinis into chunks. Chop the carrots. Finely chop the onion. Heat the oil in a saucepan (over which a steamer, metal sieve or colander will fit). Add the onion, carrots, garlic and spices and cook gently for 1 minute, stirring occasionally.

Add the tomato purée, bay leaf, eggplant, zucchinis and chickpeas. Stir in the stock. Cover and bring to a boil, then uncover and boil rapidly for 8 minutes.

Meanwhile, fork the couscous to break up any lumps and spread in a steamer, metal sieve or colander lined with a double layer of cheesecloth.

Place the couscous container over the cooking vegetables. Cover and cook for 5 minutes or until the vegetables are tender, the sauce is well reduced and the couscous is piping hot. Check the seasoning.

Spoon the couscous into a warmed serving dish and fork through. Pile the vegetables and juices on top. Garnish with plenty of chopped parsley.

Roasted Eggplant with Flatbread

CALORIES PER SERVING: 265

Serves 4 | Preparation time: 30 minutes, plus resting time | Cooking time: 55 minutes

This spicy Middle Eastern–style salad is served with unleavened homemade bread.
If you don't have time to make your own bread, serve with lightly toasted pita bread.

2 large eggplants, each
   about 12oz (350g)
4 tbsp olive oil
2 garlic cloves
1 onion
4 ripe plum tomatoes
¼ tsp turmeric
½ tsp ground cilantro
a pinch of ground
   cinnamon
a pinch of cayenne
   pepper
grated zest and juice of
   ½ lemon
2 tbsp chopped cilantro
salt and pepper
cilantro sprigs, to
   garnish

for the bread
2 tbsp (25g) bread flour,
   plus extra for rolling
   out
2 tbsp (25g) all-purpose
   flour
2 tbsp (15g) fine
   cornmeal
sesame and cumin
   seeds, for sprinkling
olive oil, for brushing

Preheat the oven to 450°F/230°C. Halve the eggplants lengthwise, then score a criss-cross pattern over the cut surface. Sprinkle with 2 teaspoons of salt and set aside for 30 minutes. Rinse thoroughly and pat dry.

Place the eggplants in a roasting tin and brush the cut surfaces liberally with 2 tablespoons of the oil. Roast in the oven for 45–50 minutes until browned and soft, brushing occasionally with more oil. Allow to cool slightly.

Meanwhile, finely chop the garlic and onion. Immerse the tomatoes in boiling water for 30 seconds, then remove and peel; dice the flesh. Heat the remaining oil in a frying pan, add the garlic and onion and fry for 5 minutes. Add the tomatoes, spices and lemon zest, fry for 1 minute, then cover and simmer for 5 minutes. Stir in lemon juice to taste. Remove from the heat and set aside to cool.

Sift the flour, cornmeal and ¼ teaspoon of salt into a bowl and work in 3 tablespoons of warm water to form a firm dough. Knead lightly, divide into four pieces and place on a floured plate. Cover with plastic wrap and let rest for 30 minutes.

Brush a griddle or heavy-based frying pan liberally with oil. Roll out each piece of dough on a well-floured surface to a thin round about 3mm thick. Sprinkle with sesame and cumin seeds and roll firmly. Cook the breads, one at a time, on the heated griddle for 1 minute each side until speckled brown.

Serve the eggplants with the sauce on top, garnished with cilantro and accompanied by the warm bread.

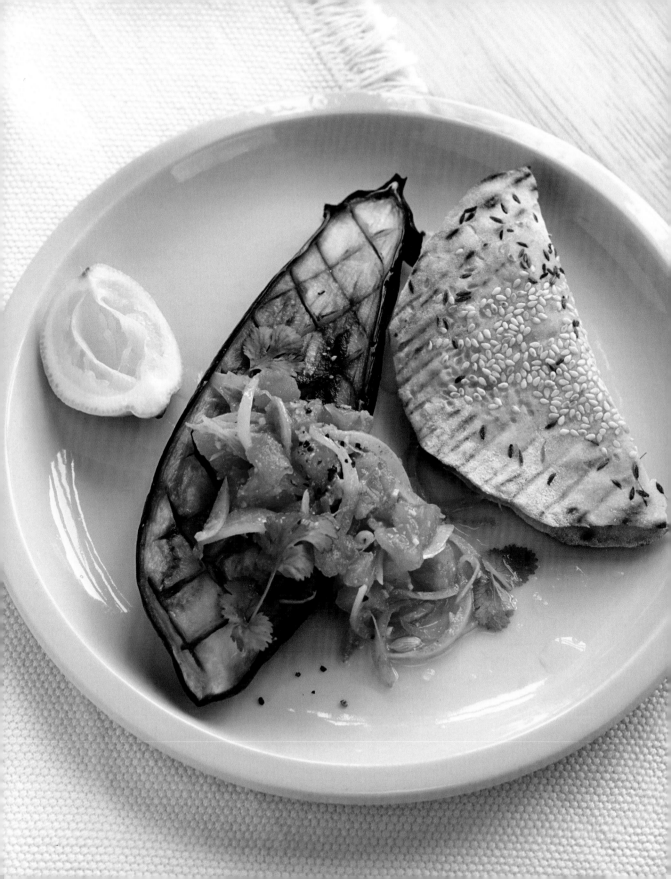

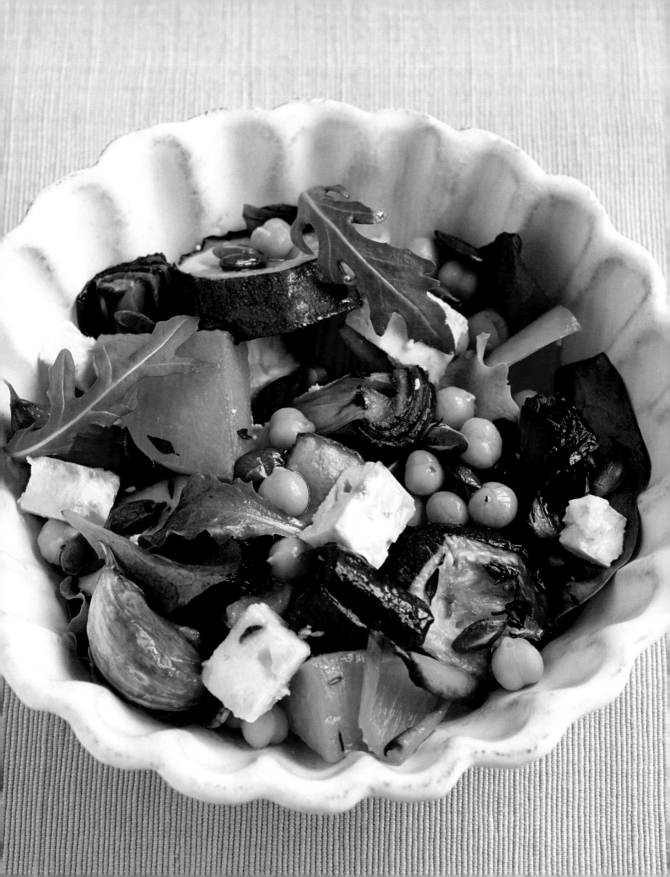

Hearty Cheese and Vegetable Salad

CALORIES PER SERVING: 268

Serves 2 | Preparation time: 10 minutes | Cooking time: 30–35 minutes

A very filling salad packed with texture and flavor—the seeds add a lovely crunch
and the cheese is deliciously creamy.

½ butternut squash,
    peeled and chopped
1 red onion, roughly
    chopped
1 zucchini, sliced into
    chunks
½ yellow pepper,
    deseeded and
    chopped into large
    pieces
2 garlic cloves,
    unpeeled
2 tsp olive oil
4 thyme sprigs
3.5oz (100g) mixed
    salad greens
1 tsp pumpkin seeds,
    toasted
3.5oz (100g) reduced-
    fat feta cheese,
    chopped
2oz (50g) canned
    chickpeas, drained
2 tsp red wine vinegar
salt and pepper

Preheat the oven to 400°F/200°C. Put all the vegetables
and the garlic in a roasting pan. Drizzle 1 teaspoon of the oil
over the vegetables then pour ¾c (200ml) water into the
bottom of the pan. Scatter over the thyme sprigs. Season
well with salt and pepper, toss everything together and roast
for 30–35 minutes, until tender.

Put the salad leaves in a large bowl with the pumpkin seeds,
cheese and chickpeas.

Whisk together the remaining oil and vinegar, and season
with salt and pepper. Add the roasted vegetables to the
salad greens, then drizzle on the dressing. Toss together and
serve.

Mixed Bean Chili

CALORIES PER SERVING: 270

Serves 6 | Preparation time: 20 minutes, plus soaking time | Cooking time: 2½–3 hours

A low-calorie version of a traditional Mexican chili. Make a big batch and freeze it for up to three months. You can use canned instead of dried beans. You will need one 15oz (425g) can of each. Rinse thoroughly and add 15 minutes before the end of the cooking time.

⅔c (125g) dried red kidney beans (or see above)

⅔c (125g) dried black-eyed peas (or see above)

1 red onion

3 garlic cloves

2–3 dried hot red chiles

25oz (700g) mixed vegetables, such as carrots, potatoes, peppers, eggplants

4 tbsp olive oil

1 tbsp mild paprika

1 tbsp tomato purée

2 tsp cumin seeds

2 bay leaves

1 cinnamon stick

1 x 15oz (400g) can chopped tomatoes

1 tbsp lime or lemon juice

a large handful of cilantro

salt and pepper

Put the dried beans in separate bowls and pour on enough cold water to cover. Leave to soak overnight.

The next day, drain the beans, put them in separate pans and cover with cold water. Boil rapidly for 10 minutes, then lower the heat. Simmer until just tender: the red kidney beans will take 1–1½ hours; the black-eyed peas 1½ hours. Add salt toward the end of the cooking time. Drain and rinse.

Finely chop the onion. Crush the garlic. Crumble the chiles, removing the seeds if a milder flavor is preferred. Peel and cut the vegetables into fairly large chunks.

Heat half of the oil in a large saucepan. Add the onion, half the garlic and half the chile. Cook, stirring, for about 5 minutes, until the onion is softened. Add the paprika, tomato purée and cumin seeds and cook, stirring, for 2 minutes. Add the bay leaves, cinnamon stick, beans and prepared vegetables, stirring to coat in the onion mixture. Cook for 2 minutes, then add the tomatoes and about ⅔c (150ml) water. Bring to the boil, lower the heat and simmer for 45 minutes to 1 hour, until the vegetables are tender. If the mixture begins to stick, add a little extra water. About halfway through cooking, taste and add more chiles if necessary.

Meanwhile, whisk together the rest of the oil, lime or lemon juice and garlic. Roughly chop the cilantro and stir into the oil mixture. Leave to stand while the chili is cooking. When the chili is ready, stir in the cilantro mixture and check the seasoning.

Beef Satay

CALORIES PER SERVING: 273

Serves 2 | Preparation time: 30 minutes, plus freezing and marinating time | Cooking time: 30 minutes

This is a delicious Thai treat. Strips of beef are marinated for several hours, threaded onto bamboo skewers and grilled until charred and tender. They are served with a peanut dipping sauce and cubes of chilled cooked rice, which provide a cool, refreshing balance to the spicy beef. Prepare the day before so the flavors have time to mingle.

6oz (175g) fillet steak
1 garlic clove
½in (1cm) piece fresh
    ginger root, peeled
1 tbsp dark soy sauce
1 tbsp sweet sherry
½ tbsp rice or wine
    vinegar
1 tsp sesame oil
¼ tsp chili powder

for the rice cubes
1oz (25g) jasmine rice
salt

for the peanut sauce
1 tbsp chopped
    unsalted peanuts
a good pinch of
    crushed chili flakes
½ garlic clove, crushed
2 tsp dark soy sauce
2 tsp lime juice
½ tsp honey
1oz (25g) coconut
    cream

Place the beef in the freezer for 15 minutes until firm. This will make it easier to slice.

Using a sharp knife, slice the beef across the grain into thin strips. Place in a shallow non-reactive dish. Crush the garlic and grate the ginger; place in a bowl with the soy sauce, sherry, vinegar, sesame oil and chili powder. Pour over the beef, stir well, cover and leave to marinate in a cool place for 2–4 hours.

Cook the rice in boiling salted water for 15 minutes until very soft. Drain and refresh under cold water. Drain thoroughly. Press the rice into a small oiled dish and smooth the surface. Cover and chill in the fridge until required.

Preheat the grill to medium. Remove the beef from the marinade and thread onto bamboo skewers in a zigzag fashion. Place the beef skewers on the grill rack and grill as close to the heat as possible for 4–5 minutes until tender, turning halfway through cooking.

Meanwhile make the peanut sauce. Put the peanuts, chili flakes, garlic, soy sauce, lime juice and honey in a small pan and heat gently. Add the creamed coconut and 3 tbsp (50ml) water and cook over a gentle heat, stirring, until smooth. Remove from the heat. Unmold the rice and cut into cubes. Serve the beef satay with the peanut dipping sauce and rice cubes.

Grilled Prosciutto with Figs

CALORIES PER SERVING: 280

Serves 4 | Preparation time: 5 minutes | Cooking time: 5–10 minutes

This is a summery dish that should be made with very plump and sweet figs. The prosciutto is cooked but still juicy, while the figs are roasted until warm and caramelized.

8 fresh ripe figs

2 tbsp olive oil, for basting

12 thin slices of prosciutto

2 tbsp extra virgin olive oil, to drizzle

crushed black peppercorns

2oz (50g) Parmesan cheese shavings

Stand each fig upright. Using a sharp knife, cut a cross through each top, leaving the base of each fig intact. Ease the figs open and brush with olive oil.

Heat a griddle and when very hot, add the figs, cut-side down, and cook for 5–10 minutes until hot and golden brown, turning once. Alternatively, place under a preheated searing-hot broiler and broil until browning and hot all the way through.

While the figs are cooking, place half the slices of prosciutto on the griddle and cook for 2–3 minutes until they start to crisp. Remove and keep warm while cooking the remaining prosciutto. (Alternatively place under a very hot grill.)

Arrange 3 slices of prosciutto and 2 figs on each warmed serving plate. Drizzle with extra virgin olive oil and season with plenty of crushed black pepper. Scatter the Parmesan shavings on top.

Chile Chicken Wrap

CALORIES PER SERVING: 316

Serves 2 │ Preparation time: 10 minutes │ Cooking time: 3 minutes

This is a perfect quick lunch that can be packed into a lunchbox and taken to work. It's a great way of making use of leftovers, but you can also use slices of lean roasted chicken.

1 tsp vegetable oil

3.5oz (100g) leftover
    roasted chicken,
    skin removed and
    shredded

½ red chile, chopped

½in (1cm) piece
    fresh ginger root,
    chopped

1 garlic clove, sliced

juice of ½ lime

1 tsp dark soy sauce

2 tsp sesame oil

2oz (50g) bean sprouts

1 carrot, grated

2oz (50g) spinach

2 tortillas

salt and pepper

Heat the vegetable oil in a non-stick frying pan or wok and add the chicken, chile, ginger and garlic. Cook for 2–3 minutes until the chicken starts to turn golden and the garlic is cooked, but not brown.

Whisk together the lime juice, soy sauce and sesame oil. Season with salt and pepper to taste.

Divide the bean sprouts, grated carrot and spinach between two tortillas, then top with the chicken. Drizzle the dressing on top, roll up and dig in!

Mexican Chicken

CALORIES PER SERVING: 325

Serves 6 | Preparation time: 30 minutes, plus marinating time | Cooking time: 15 minutes

This Mexican-style dish is bright and colorful—use different colored peppers for maximum effect. Make a big batch and keep it in the fridge to serve with salads or tortillas with guacamole and salsa.

3 onions
2–3 hot chiles
2 garlic cloves, crushed
2 tbsp chopped cilantro
grated zest and juice of
    2 limes
6 x 5oz (150g) skinless
    chicken breasts
8 red, yellow or orange
    peppers (or a
    mixture)
1–2 tbsp olive oil
salt and pepper
cilantro leaves, to
    garnish

Peel and halve the onions, leaving most of the root end attached so that they will hold their shape during cooking. Cut each half into wedges, working from the root end to the top. Slice the chiles, discarding the seeds if a milder flavor is preferred.

Put the garlic, onions, chiles, cilantro, lime zest and juice in a shallow dish and mix thoroughly. Cut the chicken into large pieces and add to the dish. Stir well, cover and leave to marinate in a cool place for at least 1 hour or overnight.

Halve the peppers and remove the cores and seeds, then cut into wedges.

Heat the oil in a heavy-based frying pan. Remove the chicken and onions from the marinade with a slotted spoon, reserving the marinade. Add the chicken and onions to the pan and cook, turning, over high heat until thoroughly browned on the outside. Remove the chicken from the pan.

Add the peppers to the pan and cook, turning, over high heat for about 5 minutes until the onions and peppers are softened.

Return the chicken to the pan, add the marinade, lower the heat and cook for about 5 minutes, stirring occasionally, or until the chicken is cooked through.

Season with salt and pepper, to taste, and sprinkle with the cilantro leaves.

Pasta with Two-Tomato Sauce

340

CALORIES PER SERVING: 340 if using regular pasta; 328 if using whole wheat pasta

Serves 6 | Preparation time: 15 minutes | Cooking time: 35–40 minutes

Made with fresh tomatoes and enriched with sun-dried tomato paste, this sauce makes a substantial meal served with pasta. Full-flavored, fresh, ripe tomatoes give the best result but canned plum tomatoes are a better choice than under-ripe or flavorless fresh ones. Make a large batch and freeze.

2 tbsp (30g) butter
1 small onion, chopped
2 garlic cloves, chopped
2¼lb (1kg) ripe tomatoes, preferably plum, or two x 24oz (400g) cans plum tomatoes with their juice
3 tbsp sun-dried tomato paste (see note)
2 oregano sprigs
14oz (400g) dried fusilli, conchiglie or penne
1oz (25g) freshly grated Parmesan cheese
salt and pepper
2 tbsp chopped flat-leaf parsley, to garnish

To prepare the sauce, melt the butter in a saucepan, add the onion and garlic, and cook over low heat for about 15 minutes while preparing the tomatoes. Add 2 tablespoons of water if the onions look like they're drying out.

If using fresh tomatoes, first skin them. Immerse in a bowl of boiling water for 30 seconds, then drain and refresh under cold running water. Peel away the skins. Quarter the tomatoes, discard the seeds, then roughly chop the flesh. If using canned plum tomatoes, chop them roughly.

Add the tomatoes to the onion and garlic mixture together with the sun-dried tomato paste and oregano sprigs. Cook, uncovered, over a low heat for 25–30 minutes, stirring occasionally, until the sauce is thick and pulpy.

Meanwhile, cook the pasta in a large pan of boiling salted water until al dente or according to the packet instructions. Drain thoroughly in a colander.

Discard the oregano and season the sauce with salt and pepper, to taste. Add the pasta and toss well to mix. Serve at once, topped with the Parmesan and chopped parsley.

Note: You can buy sun-dried tomato paste, but it's also very easy to make. Use a food processor to purée the contents of a jar of sun-dried tomatoes in oil. Return the paste to the empty jar and store in the refrigerator until required.

Chicken, Potato and Spinach Frittata

CALORIES PER SERVING: 345

Serves 4 | Preparation time: 10 minutes | Cooking time: 20 minutes

For this tempting frittata, choose low-starch potatoes like Yukon Gold or fingerling potatoes, which hold their shape when sautéed, and use a heavy-based frying pan to cook the frittata, or it will stick.

1lb (450g) low-starch
   potatoes
2 onions
8oz (220g) cooked
   chicken or turkey
4 tbsp olive oil
1 garlic clove, crushed
a handful of baby
   spinach leaves
freshly grated nutmeg,
   to taste
5 large eggs, beaten
salt and pepper

Peel the potatoes and cut into 1in (2.5cm) chunks. Cut the onions in half, then slice. Cut the chicken or turkey into bite-size pieces.

Heat half of the oil in a heavy-based, preferably non-stick, frying pan. Add the potatoes, onions and garlic. Cook over high heat until the vegetables are tinged with brown. Reduce the heat and continue cooking, stirring occasionally, until the potatoes are cooked. If the mixture starts to stick, add a little more oil.

When the potatoes are cooked, add the chicken or turkey and cook over high heat for 5 minutes or until the chicken is heated through. Add the spinach and cook until wilted, then season with salt, pepper and nutmeg.

Add a little extra oil to coat the bottom of the pan if necessary. Heat for 1 minute, then add the beaten eggs. Continue cooking over high heat for about 2 minutes, to set the egg at the bottom, then lower the heat and cook until the egg at the top is just set.

Remove the pan from the heat. Using an offset spatula, carefully loosen the frittata around the edge. Invert a plate over the pan, then turn the plate and pan over to release the frittata onto the plate. Slide the frittata back into the pan and cook for 1–2 minutes more.

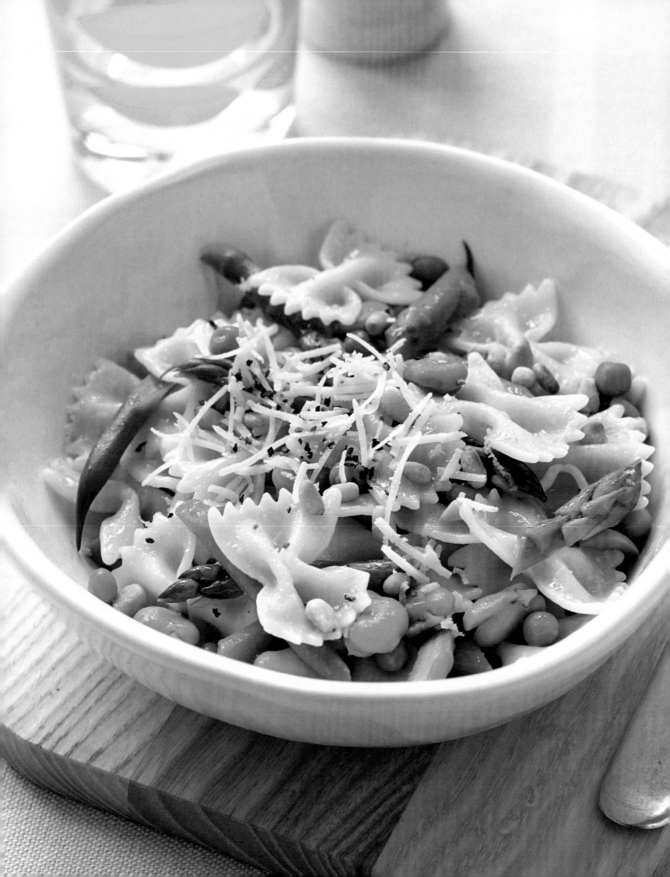

Pasta Primavera

CALORIES PER SERVING: 348 per serving; 339 if using whole wheat pasta

Serves 2 │ Preparation time: 10 minutes │ Cooking time: 20 minutes

A healthy pasta dish that's chock-full of fresh green spring vegetables. The pine nuts add a subtle creaminess to this very filling lunch.

3.5oz (100g) farfalle
1 tsp olive oil
1 garlic clove, sliced
4.5oz (125g) asparagus tips, halved
2.5oz (75g) fine green beans, halved
3.5oz (100g) shelled and skinned fava beans
2 tbsp (50g) peas
zest and juice of ½ lemon
2 tsp extra virgin olive oil
3½ tsp (10g) pine nuts, toasted
0.5oz (10g) freshly grated Parmesan cheese
salt and pepper

Cook the pasta in a large pan of boiling water according to the packet instructions.

Meanwhile, in a large frying pan, heat the olive oil and cook the garlic for 1 minute. Add the vegetables and toss to coat in the garlic. Add a ladleful of the pasta cooking water, put the lid on and allow the vegetables to steam for 5–7 minutes until just tender.

Drain the pasta, leaving a little of the cooking water clinging to it. Add the lemon zest and juice to the vegetables, season and drizzle over the extra virgin olive oil. Stir to mix.

Add the vegetables to the pasta, then divide between two plates. Scatter the pine nuts and Parmesan on top.

Kleftiko

CALORIES PER SERVING: 350

Serves 4 | Preparation time: 15 minutes, plus marinating time | Cooking time: 2–2½ hours

Kleftiko—or "robber's lamb" as it is literally translated—is a traditional Greek recipe in which the lamb is seasoned with lemon and oregano and then cooked in a covered dish until meltingly tender.

8 lamb loin chops, or
    4 leg steaks (with
    bone)
2 lemons
1 tbsp dried oregano
2 tbsp olive oil
2 onions
2 bay leaves
⅔c (150ml) dry white
    wine
⅔c (150ml) stock
salt and pepper
lemon wedges, to serve

Place the lamb in a single layer in a shallow dish. Squeeze the juice from the lemons into a small bowl or cup and add the oregano, salt and pepper. Sprinkle the mixture over the meat and leave to marinate in a cool place for at least 4 hours, preferably overnight.

Preheat the oven to 325°F/160°C. Heat the oil in a large frying pan. Lift the lamb chops out of the marinade and add them to the pan. Cook over high heat, turning until well browned on all sides, then transfer to a shallow earthenware casserole.

Peel and slice the onions and add to the lamb, together with the bay leaves, wine and stock. Pour in any remaining marinade and season with pepper.

Cover the dish with foil. Bake in the oven for 2–2½ hours until the lamb is tender, removing the foil for the last 20 minutes to brown the meat.

Before serving, carefully skim off any excess fat. Serve the meat with the juices spooned over with lemon wedges on the side.

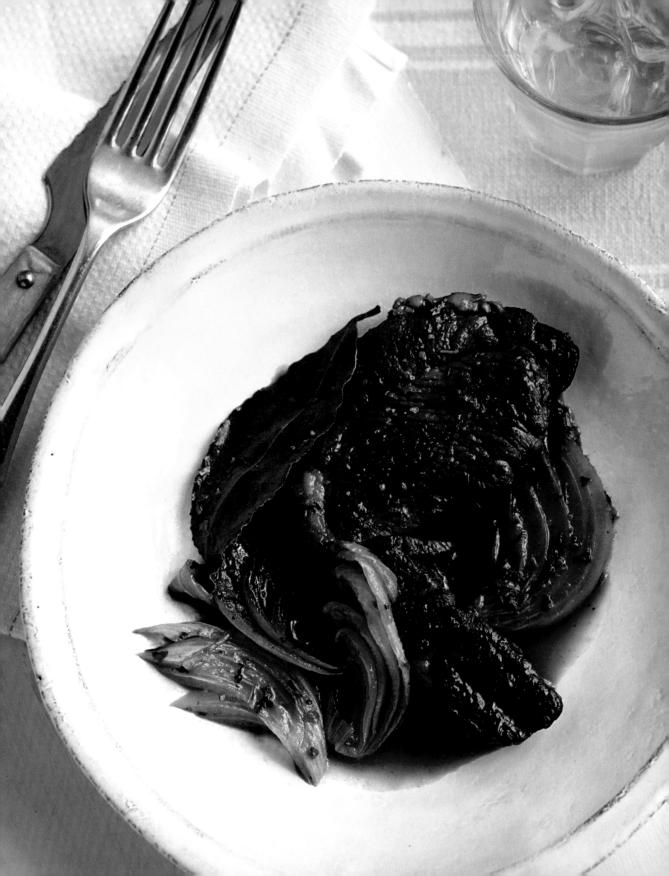

Stuffed Sardines

CALORIES PER SERVING: 365

Serves 4 │ Preparation time: 25 minutes │ Cooking time: 10 minutes

Fresh sardines are stuffed with a sweet and savory mixture of pine nuts, parsley and raisins, then rolled and baked until tender.

16 fresh sardines
⅓c (50g) pine nuts,
   toasted
2oz (50g) raisins
3 tbsp chopped flat-leaf
   parsley
finely grated zest and
   juice of 1 orange
⅓c (100ml) olive oil
salt and pepper

Preheat the oven to 350°F/180°C. Scrape the scales from the sardines if necessary, then cut off the heads. Slit open the bellies and clean the insides under cold running water. Lay flesh-side down on a cutting board. Slide your thumb along the backbone, pressing firmly to release the flesh along its length. Take hold of the backbone at the head end and lift it out; the fish should now be open like a book.

For the stuffing, mix together the pine nuts, raisins, parsley, orange zest, and salt and pepper, to taste. Place a spoonful of stuffing on the flesh side of each fish. Roll up from the head end and secure with a toothpick if necessary.

Place the stuffed sardines in an oiled ovenproof dish into which they fit snugly. It is important that the sardines are tightly packed together. Pour the orange juice and olive oil on top. Season with salt and pepper and bake for about 10 minutes.

Note: The cooking time will vary depending on the type of baking dish used. The sardines will cook more quickly in a thin metal baking pan than in a terracotta baking dish, for example. Avoid using frozen sardines as they have a disappointing flavor.

Pasta and Chickpea Soup with Arugula Pesto

CALORIES PER SERVING: 370

Serves 6 | Preparation time: 25 minutes | Cooking time: 1 hour

This soup's pesto is made with peppery arugula rather than the usual basil, giving a cleaner taste to the finished soup. Make a large batch and then freeze before you add the pesto.

4 ripe tomatoes
3 tbsp olive oil
1 onion, chopped
2 garlic cloves, finely
    chopped
1 leek, trimmed and sliced
1 tbsp chopped rosemary
1 x 14oz (400g) can of
    chickpeas
5c (1.2 liters) vegetable stock
1 zucchini, diced
4.5oz (125g) shelled peas
4.5oz (125g) green beans,
    halved
4.5oz (125g) shelled and
    skinned fava beans
4.5oz (50g) small pasta shells
2 tbsp chopped flat-leaf
    parsley
salt and pepper

for the arugula pesto
4.5oz (50g) arugula
1 garlic clove, peeled
1 tbsp capers, rinsed and
    drained
1 tbsp chopped flat-leaf
    parsley
0.5oz (15g) pine nuts, toasted
0.5oz (15g) freshly grated
    Parmesan cheese
5 tbsp extra virgin olive oil

Immerse the tomatoes in a bowl of boiling water for 30 seconds, then remove with a slotted spoon and peel away the skins. Chop the tomato flesh.

Heat the oil in a large saucepan, add the onion, garlic, leek and rosemary and fry gently for 10 minutes until softened but not colored. Add the chickpeas with their liquid, the stock and tomatoes. Bring to a boil, cover and simmer for 30 minutes.

Meanwhile make the arugula pesto. Wash and dry the arugula leaves and chop roughly. Place in a grinder or food processor and add the garlic, capers, parsley, pine nuts and Parmesan. Purée to form a fairly smooth paste, then stir in the oil and season with salt and pepper, to taste.

Add the zucchini, peas and beans to the soup. Return to a boil and simmer for another 10 minutes. Add the pasta and parsley and cook for 6–8 minutes until the pasta is al dente. Check and adjust the seasoning with salt and pepper.

Serve the soup in warmed bowls with the arugula pesto spooned into the middle.

Hearty Stew

CALORIES PER SERVING: 390

Serves 6 | Preparation time: 20 minutes | Cooking time: 1 hour

This satisfying stew relies on a good mix of root vegetables to bolster up the chicken flavor. The split lentils thicken the liquid and heighten the robust feel of the meal. It's a great dish to freeze and have on standby.

1 x 3lb (1.4kg) chicken
  (or chicken pieces)
2 tbsp all-purpose flour
2 tbsp olive oil
2 onions
2 parsnips
2 large carrots
2 large potatoes
4oz (125g) split red
  lentils
2 bay leaves
2 garlic cloves
1 x 14oz (400g) can of
  black-eyed peas or
  red kidney beans,
  drained
2 zucchinis, sliced
3 tbsp chopped flat-leaf
  parsley
1 tbsp chopped fresh
  chives
salt and pepper

Butcher the chicken into even-sized pieces. Sprinkle the chicken with flour and season with salt and pepper.

Heat the oil in a Dutch oven and cook the chicken in batches until well browned on all sides. Remove from the pan and set aside.

Meanwhile, roughly chop the onions. Peel the parsnips, carrots and potatoes; cut them all into chunks. Add a little extra oil to the pan if necessary and cook the vegetables until lightly browned.

Return the chicken to the pan and add the lentils, bay leaves, garlic and 4c (900ml) water. Cover with a tight-fitting lid and simmer gently, stirring occasionally, for 45 minutes or until the chicken is tender and the lentils are soft and mushy.

Rinse the beans and add to the pan with the zucchini. Season to taste with salt and pepper. Cook for another 15 minutes or until the zucchinis are just tender and the beans are heated through. If the sauce is too thin, retrieve a few spoonfuls of vegetables, mash them with a potato masher and return to the stew to thicken it slightly. Sprinkle with the chopped parsley and chives.

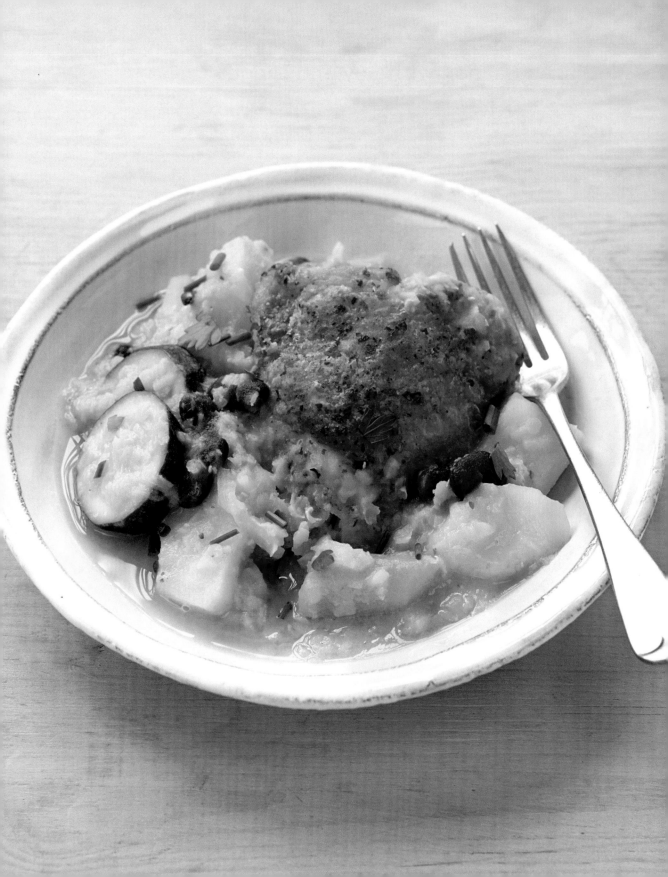

Glazed Salmon with Soy and Ginger

CALORIES PER SERVING: 406

Serves 4 | Preparation time: 20 minutes | Cooking time: 10 minutes

Based on the Japanese teriyaki style of cooking, salmon fillets are marinated in a well-flavored mixture that makes a shiny glaze once the fish is grilled.

2½in (6cm) piece fresh
    ginger root
1 garlic clove, peeled
6 tbsp light soy sauce
8 tbsp mirin (Japanese
    rice wine) or sweet
    sherry
1 tbsp soft brown sugar
4 x 6oz (175g) salmon
    fillets
7oz (200g) bok choy

Crush the ginger and garlic using a pestle and mortar until the juices start to run. Then, using your hands, squeeze out as much of the juice as possible into a shallow dish, taking care to exclude any solid pieces of ginger or garlic (as these would burn during cooking and spoil the effect).

Put the soy sauce, mirin and sugar into a small saucepan and dissolve over low heat, then bring to a boil, stirring all the time. Boil for about 5 minutes until the mixture is slightly reduced and syrupy. Pour on to the ginger juice and leave to cool completely.

Add the fish to the dish and turn to coat with the marinade on all sides. Leave to marinate in a cool place for 30 minutes to 1 hour.

Preheat a grill pan to high. Thread the fish onto two long skewers. Thoroughly oil the grill and lay the fish in the pan, skin-side down. Grill for about 6–8 minutes or until the fish flakes easily when tested with a fork, brushing frequently during cooking with the excess marinade. If the salmon appears to be overcooking on the surface but not cooking underneath, lower the position of the grill pan rather than turn the fish over.

Steam the bok choy in a pan with a splash of water until tender. Serve with the salmon.

Mushroom and Parmesan Risotto

CALORIES PER SERVING: 420

Serves 4 │ Preparation time: 15 minutes │ Cooking time: 20 minutes

This is a wonderfully warming meal for a cold night. Make sure you pare the lemon rind in one large piece, so it's easy to remove.

1 lemon
6oz (175g) button
   mushrooms
6oz (175g) green beans
8oz (225g) broccoli
   florets
2 tbsp olive oil
1 medium onion, finely
   chopped
2c (350g) Arborio rice
optional: a pinch of
   saffron threads
4 tbsp dry white wine
3c (750ml) vegetable
   stock
salt and pepper
1 tbsp finely shaved
   Parmesan cheese, to
   serve

Finely pare the rind from the lemon, using a vegetable peeler, then squeeze the juice. Wipe the mushrooms clean with a damp cloth, then slice.

Trim the green beans and cut in half lengthways. Blanch the broccoli and beans together in boiling salted water for 3–4 minutes. Drain and refresh under cold running water.

Heat the oil in a heavy-based saucepan or Dutch oven and cook the onion gently for 2–3 minutes until beginning to soften. Stir in the rice and saffron, if using. Season well with salt and pepper and pour in the wine. Add the pared lemon rind, 2 tablespoons of lemon juice and the stock. Bring to a boil, stirring.

Cover and simmer the risotto for 5 minutes. Stir in the mushrooms, broccoli and green beans. Re-cover and simmer for another 5 minutes, or until the rice is tender and most of the liquid is absorbed.

Discard the lemon rind and transfer the risotto to warmed serving plates. Top with slivers of Parmesan cheese and serve at once.

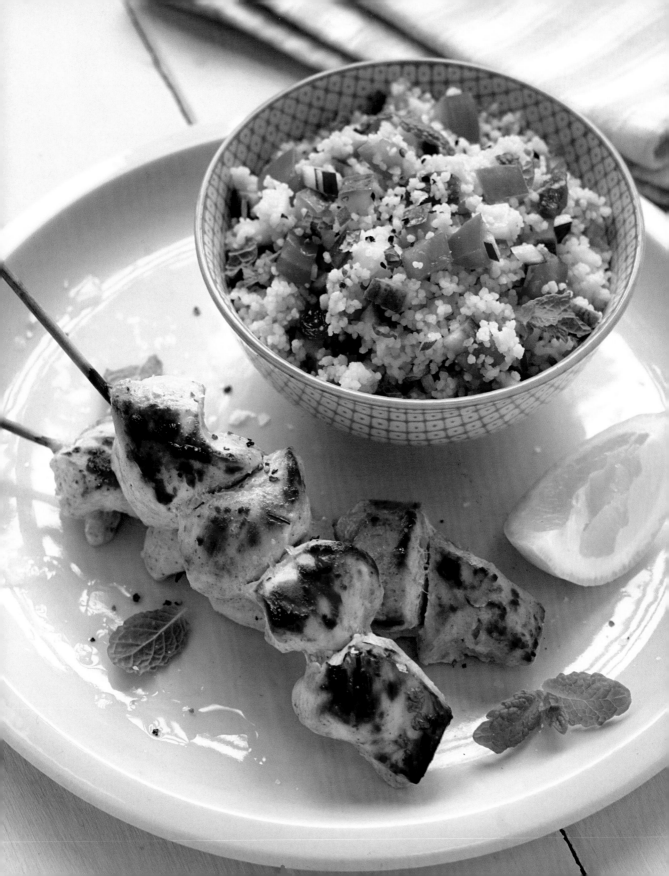

Tandoori Chicken with Minted Couscous

CALORIES PER SERVING: 440

Serves 6 │ Preparation time: 20 minutes, plus marinating time │ Cooking time: 20 minutes

The dressing for the couscous is sweet and balances the tangy chicken beautifully. Make enough to serve six and have the rest for lunch or dinner the following day.

6 x 4.5oz (125g) skinless chicken breasts
9oz (275ml) Greek-style yogurt
2 garlic cloves, crushed
1in (2.5cm) piece fresh ginger root, peeled and grated
finely grated zest and juice of ½ lemon
2 tsp hot curry paste
1 tsp paprika
½ tsp salt
8oz (225g) quick-cook couscous
4 ripe tomatoes, deseeded and diced
1 small red onion, finely chopped
lemon wedges and mint sprigs, to serve

for the dressing
juice of 2 lemons
2 tbsp (25g) baker's sugar
1oz (25g) mint leaves
4.5oz (125g) cucumber
2oz (50g) golden raisins
4 tbsp extra virgin olive oil
salt and pepper

Wash and dry the chicken breast fillets and cut into 1in (2.5cm) cubes. Put the yogurt in a large bowl with the garlic, ginger, lemon zest and juice, curry paste, paprika and salt. Add the chicken pieces, toss well to coat and leave to marinate in a cool place overnight.

The next day, wash the couscous to moisten and place in a cheesecloth-lined steamer. Place over a pan of simmering water, cover with a tight-fitting lid and cook for 5–6 minutes until fluffy.

Meanwhile, prepare the dressing. Put the lemon juice and sugar in a saucepan and heat gently until dissolved. Stir in the remaining ingredients, season with salt and pepper, to taste, and remove from the heat.

Transfer the couscous to a large bowl, add the dressing and stir with a fork until evenly mixed. Add the tomatoes and onion to the couscous, season to taste and set aside.

Preheat the grill. Remove the chicken from the marinade and thread onto 6 skewers. Grill for 10–15 minutes, turning frequently, until the chicken is charred on the outside and cooked through. Leave to cool.

Spoon the couscous onto individual plates and top with the skewers. Garnish with lemon wedges and mint.

Note: If using bamboo skewers, pre-soak in cold water for 30 minutes to prevent them scorching on the grill.

Penne with Olives, Anchovy and Chili

CALORIES PER SERVING: 445

Serves 6 │ Preparation time: 10 minutes │ Cooking time: 10 minutes

Use olives from the delicatessen that have been marinating in flavored oils. They are usually far more delicious than olives found in jars and can be much cheaper. You won't need to add salt to this dish, as the ingredients themselves are naturally salty.

14oz (400g) dried
   penne
2 garlic cloves
2oz (50g) anchovies in
   olive oil
½ tsp dried chili flakes
2 tbsp chopped flat-leaf
   parsley
8 oz (230g) pitted mixed
   black and green olives
4 tbsp extra virgin olive oil
2 tbsp freshly grated
   Parmesan cheese,
   plus extra to serve
pepper

Bring a large saucepan of salted water to a boil. Add the pasta and cook until al dente, or according to the package instructions.

Meanwhile, thinly slice the garlic cloves. Place in a saucepan with the anchovies and their oil. Add the chili flakes and cook over fairly high heat for 2–3 minutes, stirring to break up the anchovies with a wooden spoon; do not allow the garlic to brown. Stir in the parsley and remove from the heat.

Transfer the contents of the pan to a food processor and add the olives and olive oil. Process for a few seconds to make a coarse paste. Season with pepper, to taste.

When the pasta is cooked, drain thoroughly in a colander. Return to the saucepan and add the olive mixture and freshly grated Parmesan. Toss well to coat the pasta. Serve immediately, topped with a sprinkling of Parmesan shavings.

Lamb with Potato

CALORIES PER SERVING: 450

Serves 2 │ Preparation time: 20 minutes │ Cooking time: 1½ hours

Use low-starch potatoes such as Yukon Gold or fingerling for this dish and don't cut them into small pieces or they will disintegrate during cooking.

1 hot red chile

1 small onion, quartered

1 garlic clove

½in (1cm) piece
fresh ginger root,
peeled and roughly
chopped

1 tbsp desiccated
coconut

10.5oz (300g) lean
boneless lamb

7oz (200g) low-starch
potatoes

1 tbsp ghee or
vegetable oil

1 tsp paprika

½ tsp ground fenugreek

½ tsp ground turmeric

1 tsp ground coriander

½ tsp tsp ground cumin

2oz (50ml) yogurt

3.5oz (100ml) meat or
vegetable stock

salt and pepper

Preheat the oven to 350°F/180°C. Chop the chile, discarding the seeds if a milder flavor is preferred. Put the onion, garlic, ginger, chile and coconut in a blender with 1 tablespoon of water and process until smooth.

Trim the meat of any excess fat and cut into 4cm cubes. Peel the potatoes and cut into large chunks.

Heat the ghee or oil in a Dutch oven, add the onion paste and cook until golden brown, stirring all the time. Add the spices and cook, stirring, over high heat for 2 minutes.

Brown the meat and potatoes in the pan over high heat, in batches if necessary, turning constantly until thoroughly browned on all sides. Lower the heat and return all the meat and potatoes to the. Add the yogurt, a spoonful at a time, stirring after each addition.

Add the stock and season liberally with salt. Bring to a boil, then reduce the heat, cover and cook in the oven for about 2 hours or until the meat is very tender.

When the meat and potatoes are tender, remove with a slotted spoon; set aside. Bring the sauce to a boil and boil steadily until the sauce is well reduced and very thick. Return the meat and potatoes to the pan and stir to coat with the sauce.

dinner

Thai Fishcakes

CALORIES PER FISCAKE: 100

Makes 10 | Preparation time: 25 minutes | Cooking time: 20 minutes

Bursting with strong flavors from the chilies, Kaffir lime leaves and lemongrass, these bear absolutely no resemblance to the traditional British fishcake! Serve them on a bed of crunchy fresh salad greens. This recipe makes 10, so freeze any you aren't planning on using immediately.

1lb (450g) white fish
    fillets, such as cod or
    haddock
4 Kaffir lime leaves
2 tbsp chopped cilantro
1 tbsp Thai fish sauce
1 tbsp lime juice
2 tbsp Thai red curry
    paste
salt and pepper
flour, for coating
vegetable oil, for
    pan-frying

to serve
mixed salad greens
shredded spring onion
1 mild red chile, sliced
lime wedges

Remove any skin and pin bones from the fish, then place the fish in a food processor or blender and work until smooth.

Finely chop the lime leaves and add to the fish with the cilantro, fish sauce, lime juice and red curry paste. Season with salt and pepper. Process until well mixed.

Using lightly floured hands, divide the mixture into 10 pieces and shape each one into a cake, about 6cm in diameter.

Fry the fishcakes in batches. Heat a ½in (1cm) depth of oil in a frying pan. Cook the fishcakes, a few at a time, for about 4 minutes each side. Drain on crumpled paper towels and keep hot while cooking the remainder.

Serve the fishcakes as soon as they are all cooked on a bed of salad greens scattered with shredded spring onion and chile slices. Serve with lime wedges.

Vegetable, Noodle and Tofu Broth

CALORIES PER SERVING: 130

Serves 4 | Preparation time: 20 minutes | Cooking time: 1¼ hours

The success of this soup depends on the quality of the stock, which is used to poach a selection of vegetables and the tofu. The following recipe makes an authentic Thai stock— make a large batch and freeze the stock to use in this or other soups.

1oz (25g) dried black or
    shiitake mushrooms
1 large carrot
2oz (50g) cauliflower florets
2oz (50g) baby corn
3.5oz (100g) plain tofu
2 tbsp dark soy sauce
1 tbsp lemon or lime juice
2oz (50g) dried egg thread
    noodles
mint leaves, to serve
chili oil, to serve

for the Thai-style stock
1 onion, roughly chopped
2 carrots, roughly chopped
2 celery sticks, roughly
    chopped
2 garlic cloves, roughly
    chopped
2 lemongrass stalks, roughly
    chopped
0.5oz (15g) fresh ginger root,
    roughly chopped
4 Kaffir lime leaves
4 cilantro roots, scrubbed
1 tsp white peppercorns
1 tsp salt

Start by making the stock. Place 5c (1.2 liters) water in a large saucepan and add the onion, carrots, celery, garlic, lemongrass and ginger. Scatter over the remaining ingredients, bring to a boil, cover and simmer over a gentle heat for 1 hour.

Put the dried mushrooms in a bowl, pour over ½c (120ml) boiling water and leave to soak for 30 minutes. Strain and reserve the liquid; chop the mushrooms.

Prepare the remaining vegetables. Cut the carrot into matchsticks; divide the cauliflower into small florets; halve the sweetcorn lengthways; set aside. Cube the tofu.

Strain the stock into a clean pan and stir in the soy sauce, lemon or lime juice and reserved mushroom liquid. Return to a boil and stir in the prepared vegetables, tofu and soaked mushrooms. Simmer for 5 minutes.

Plunge in the noodles and simmer for another 5–6 minutes until the noodles and vegetables are tender. Ladle the soup into large warmed soup bowls. Serve at once, scattered with mint leaves and drizzled with a little chili oil.

Grilled Stuffed Peppers

CALORIES PER SERVING: 135

Serves 4 │ Preparation time: 20 minutes │ Cooking time: 20 minutes

A colorful salad full of flavors evocative of the Mediterranean—smoky grilled peppers, aromatic fennel and garlic, and a sweet balsamic vinegar dressing.

2 small onions
2 red peppers
2 yellow peppers
2 garlic cloves, peeled
2 tbsp capers
1 tbsp fennel seeds
3½ tbsp olive oil
1½ tbsp balsamic
    vinegar
2 tbsp roughly torn
    flat-leaf parsley
coarse sea salt and
    pepper

Peel the onions, leaving the root end intact, and cut into quarters. Drop them into a pan of boiling water and cook for 1 minute; drain well.

Preheat the broiler to high. Halve the peppers lengthwise cutting through the stems, then core and deseed them. Arrange on a baking sheet, skin-side up, in a single layer (you may need to do this in two batches). Place the onion quarters and garlic cloves on the rack too. Broil until the pepper skins are blistered and well charred. Turn the onions and garlic as necessary, but let them char slightly too.

Place the peppers in a bowl, cover with a plate and allow to cool slightly, then peel away their skins. Arrange the peppers on a serving platter. Fill the cavities with the grilled onions and capers.

Put the fennel seeds in a dry frying pan and toast over medium heat for a few minutes until they begin to pop and release their aroma. Transfer to a mortar and pestle and coarsely grind them. Add the grilled garlic and grind to a paste. Transfer the garlic paste to a small bowl and whisk in the oil and vinegar.

Sprinkle the parsley, sea salt and pepper over the salad and spoon on the dressing. Serve at room temperature.

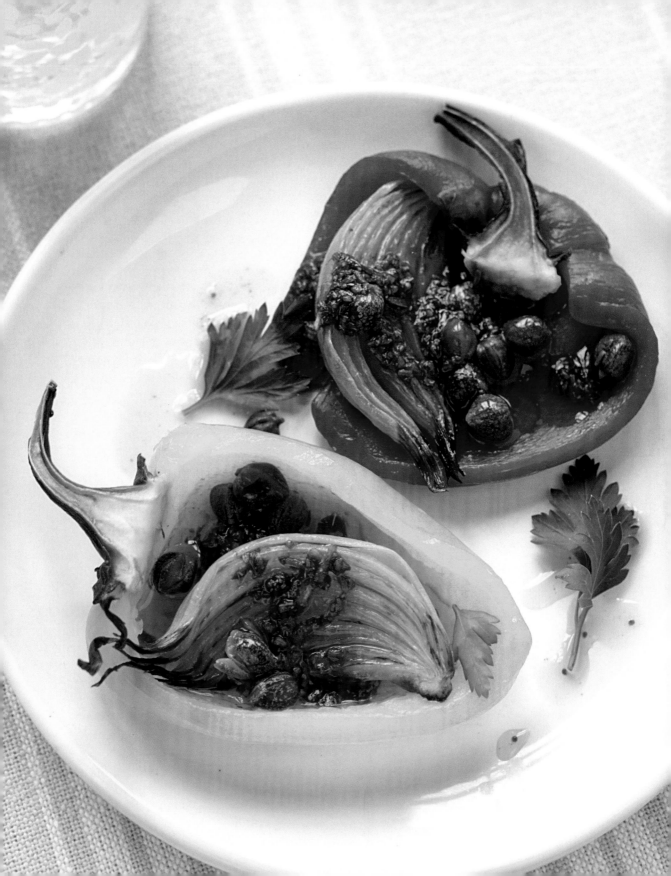

Salad of Bayonne Ham, Melon and Artichokes

CALORIES PER SERVING: 143

Serves 4 | Preparation time: 35 minutes | Cooking time: 10 minutes

In France, country or mountain hams are dried and sometimes smoked too. They are typically served in thick slices as part of a salad or *assiette de charcuterie*. Here the classic combination of salty ham and sweet juicy melon is enhanced with tender young artichoke hearts and an herb vinaigrette.

8 fresh baby artichokes
lemon juice, for
    brushing
1 tbsp olive oil
½ ripe orange-fleshed
    melon, such as
    charentais or
    cantaloupe
4 thick slices Bayonne
    ham or prosciutto
salt and pepper
mixed salad greens and
    herb sprigs, to serve

for the herb vinaigrette
2 tsp red wine vinegar
1 tsp Dijon mustard
2 tbsp olive oil
1 tbsp chopped chervil
    or tarragon

To prepare the artichokes, break off the tough outer leaves at the base until you expose a central core of pale leaves. Slice off the tough green or purple tips. Using a small, sharp knife, pare the dark green skin from the base and down the stem. Brush the cut parts with lemon juice to prevent browning. Cut into quarters and brush with lemon juice.

Heat the oil in a sauté pan or heavy-based frying pan. Add the artichokes and cook over high heat, stirring constantly, until they are just turning brown. Transfer to a bowl and allow to cool. Season with salt and pepper.

Halve the melon and scoop out the seeds. Either scoop the flesh into balls, cut into cubes or skin and slice thinly. Place the melon in the bowl with the artichokes. Toss lightly to mix.

Whisk all the ingredients for the dressing together until evenly mixed. Season with salt and pepper, to taste. Pour over the artichokes and melon and turn to coat.

Using a sharp knife, slice the ham or proscuitto into strips and add to the melon and artichokes. Arrange a few salad greens on each individual serving plate and spoon the salad on top. Garnish with herb sprigs and serve immediately.

Note: Be sure to choose a fully ripe melon. A sweet, perfumed aroma is the best indicator of ripeness. If fresh baby artichokes are unavailable, use 12 frozen prepared artichoke hearts instead; defrost thoroughly before use.

Spiced Lentil Soup

CALORIES PER SERVING: 148

Serves 2 │ Preparation time: 5 minutes │ Cooking time: 20 minutes

Sweet potato, carrots and red lentils give this warming soup a vibrant and uplifting color. The chile and spices add a touch of heat—add a little more chile if you prefer it a bit hotter.

1 sweet potato, peeled
   and chopped
1 carrot, chopped
2 tbsp split red lentils
2c (500ml) vegetable
   stock
½ red chile, chopped
¼ tsp cumin seeds
¼ tsp ground coriander
salt and pepper
a squeeze of lemon
   juice, to serve

Place the sweet potato and carrot in a saucepan. Add the red lentils, stock, chile, cumin seeds and ground coriander. Season well with salt and pepper.

Cover the pan and bring to a boil. Once it's boiling, turn the heat down low and simmer for 10 minutes, until the lentils are soft.

Purée the soup, check and adjust the seasoning with salt and pepper, and squeeze the lemon juice on top.

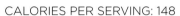

Thai Mussel Salad

CALORIES SERVING: 156

Serves 2 │ Preparation time: 25 minutes │ Cooking time: 10 minutes

Succulent mussels—fragrant with Thai flavorings—are served on a nest of vegetable ribbons and frisée. If time permits, soak the mussels in a bowl of cold water with a handful of oatmeal added for several hours before cooking to help rid them of any grit.

1 small carrot, julienned

1 small zucchini, julienned

½ small fennel bulb, finely
    sliced

1 tsp salt

9oz (250g) live mussels

1 tsp vegetable oil

2oz (50g) frisée (curly
    endive)

a handful of Thai basil leaves
    or celery leaves, to serve

for the stock

1 garlic clove, peeled

½in (1cm) fresh ginger root,
    peeled and sliced

1 Kaffir lime leaf, bruised

1 lemongrass stalk, bruised

1 red chile, bruised

½ tbsp Thai fish sauce

for the dressing

2 tbsp lime juice

1 tbsp rice wine vinegar

2½ tsp (10g) baker's sugar

½ tsp crushed red chiles

¼ tsp salt

Place the carrot, zucchini and fennel in a colander and sprinkle with the salt. Set aside to drain for 30 minutes.

In the meantime, scrub the mussels thoroughly under cold running water and pull away any straggly beards. Discard any opened mussels that do not close when tapped firmly.

Place all the stock ingredients in a saucepan with ⅔c (150ml) cold water. Bring to a boil, cover and simmer for 10 minutes, then strain into a clean pan.

Add the mussels to the stock, bring to a boil, cover and cook over high heat for 4–5 minutes or until the shells have opened. Discard any mussels that remain closed. Strain, reserving the liquid, and immediately refresh the mussels under cold running water. Drain and set aside.

Place 3 tablespoons of the reserved mussel liquid in a pan. Add the dressing ingredients, heat gently to dissolve the sugar, then keep warm.

Wash the vegetables to remove the salt and pat dry thoroughly with paper towels.

Heat the vegetable oil in a wok and fry the vegetables in batches for 2–3 minutes until golden.

Divide the frisée between serving plates, top with the vegetables and sit the mussels on top. Spoon the warm dressing on top and serve at once, garnished with Thai basil or celery leaves.

Prawns with Spinach

CALORIES PER SERVING: 162

Serves 4 | Preparation time: 25 minutes | Cooking time: 15 minutes

Fresh spinach gives this dish a wonderful vibrance and it contrasts deliciously with the creamy prawns. Most coconut milk comes in 14oz (400ml) cans, but you can freeze the remaining ¾c (200ml) for up to a month.

25oz (700g) large raw
    prawns in shells
1lb (450g) spinach
2 tbsp vegetable oil
1 medium onion, sliced
1 garlic clove, sliced
2in (5cm) piece fresh
    ginger root, peeled
    and cut into thin
    strips
2 tsp ground turmeric
1 tsp chili powder
1 tbsp black mustard
    seeds
2 tsp ground coriander
a large pinch of ground
    cloves
¾c (200ml) reduced-fat
    coconut milk
1 tbsp lime or lemon
    juice
salt

To prepare the raw prawns, remove the heads, if necessary, then peel off the shell leaving the fan-like piece at the end of the tail attached. Using a small, sharp knife, make a shallow slit along the back of each prawn and remove the dark intestinal vein. Rinse the prawns under cold running water. Drain and pat dry with paper towels.

Trim the spinach leaves and wash thoroughly in several changes of water if necessary; drain well.

Heat the oil in a large frying pan or wok. Add the onion, garlic and ginger and fry, stirring, until softened. Add the spices and cook for 2 minutes, stirring all the time.

Add the coconut milk, bring to a boil, then lower the heat and simmer for 5 minutes. Add the prawns and simmer for about 4 minutes or until they just begin to look opaque.

Add the spinach; it may be difficult to fit it all in but don't worry, it will reduce as it cooks in the steam. Cover the pan with a lid or a baking tray and cook for about 3 minutes or until the spinach is wilted; don't keep removing the lid to check during cooking or you will let the steam escape. Stir the wilted spinach into the sauce, add the lime or lemon juice and serve.

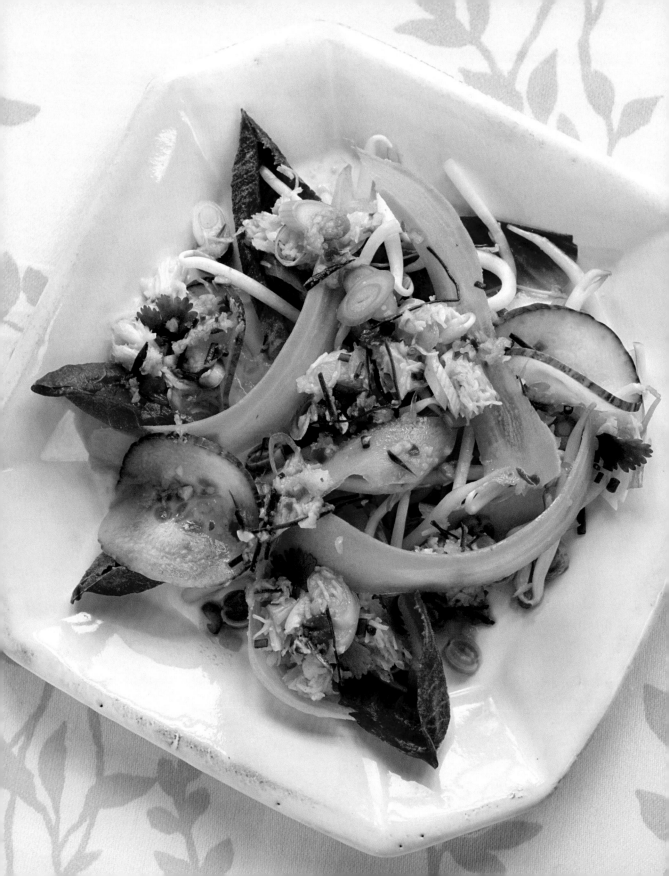

Crab Salad

CALORIES PER SERVING: 168

Serves 6 │ Preparation time: 20 minutes │ Cooking time: 3 minutes

There is nothing quite like the taste of freshly cooked crab meat and this salad is the perfect way to appreciate it. If using fresh cooked crabs, you will need two, each about 3lb (1.4kg). The dark meat is not included in this dish but it can be frozen for future use.

1lb (450g) white crab meat
6 spring onions, trimmed
2 tbsp chopped cilantro
1 tbsp chopped chives
a pinch of cayenne pepper
2 garlic cloves
1in (2.5cm) piece fresh ginger root, peeled
2 tbsp vegetable oil
2 Kaffir lime leaves, shredded
½ tsp dried crushed chili flakes
4 tbsp lime juice
1 tbsp sugar
1 tsp shrimp paste
1 tbsp Thai fish sauce or soy sauce
2 heads of radicchio or red chicory
2oz (50g) cucumber
1oz (25g) bean sprouts
1 carrot, finely sliced
lime wedges, to serve
a handful of cilantro leaves, to serve

Flake the white crab meat into shreds and place in a bowl. Finely chop the spring onions and add to the crab with the cilantro, chives and cayenne pepper. Mix gently, then cover and chill until required.

Crush the garlic and ginger together, using a pestle and mortar. Heat the oil in a small pan, add the garlic, ginger, lime leaves and chili flakes and fry over a gentle heat for 3 minutes until softened but not brown. Add the lime juice, sugar, shrimp paste and fish sauce or soy sauce. Stir well, then remove from the heat. Leave to cool.

Drizzle the cooled dressing over the crab mixture and toss lightly until evenly combined. Arrange the radicchio or chicory leaves on serving plates and spoon over the crab mixture. Thinly slice the cucumber and arrange on top of each serving with the bean sprouts and carrot. Garnish with lime wedges and cilantro leaves.

Glazed Chicken Wings

CALORIES PER SERVING: 175

Serves 4 | Preparation time: 10 minutes, plus marinating time | Cooking time: 1 hour

The spices and flavorings in this recipe make a rich glaze for the chicken wings. It is simple and quick to prepare, but the longer the wings are left to marinate, the more flavor they absorb.

12 small chicken wings
4 garlic cloves
2 tsp hot chili sauce
3 tbsp soy sauce
1 tbsp preserved stem
    ginger syrup or
    honey
1 tbsp lemon juice
1 tsp ground coriander
½ tsp ground cinnamon
2 spring onions,
    shredded, to serve
lime or lemon wedges,
    to serve

Wash and dry the chicken wings. Tuck the tip of each wing under the thickest part of the wing, forming a triangular shape. Transfer to a large shallow, non-reactive dish.

Crush the garlic and place in a bowl. Add all the remaining ingredients, mix well, then pour over the chicken wings. Toss to coat the wings thoroughly. Cover and leave to marinate in a cool place for at least 4 hours, preferably overnight.

Preheat the oven to 425°F/220°C. Transfer the chicken wings and marinade juices to a roasting pan just large enough to hold them in a single layer. Bake at the top of the oven for about an hour, basting and turning frequently until the wings are glazed and tender. The flesh should almost fall from the bone. Serve hot, with spring onion shreds and lime and/or lemon wedges.

Roasted Tomatoes with a Garlic Crust

CALORIES PER SERVING: 185

Serves 6 │ Preparation time: 15 minutes │ Cooking time: 20 minutes

In this easy adaptation of the classic stuffed tomato, flavorful cherry or other small tomatoes are baked whole under a delicious crust of chopped garlic, parsley, toasted breadcrumbs and olive oil.

6 slices day-old stale bread
6 garlic cloves
3 tbsp chopped fresh parsley, plus extra to garnish
25oz (700g) cherry tomatoes
olive oil, for basting
salt and pepper

Preheat the oven to 425˚F/220˚C. Tear up the bread and place in a food processor or blender. Process until you have fine breadcrumbs; there should be approximately ½c (125g). Place in a heavy-based frying pan and toast over moderate heat until golden.

Finely chop the garlic. Stir into the breadcrumbs with the chopped parsley and salt and pepper, to taste.

Place the tomatoes in a shallow roasting pan or dish, positioning them close together and in a single layer. Sprinkle the breadcrumbs evenly over the tomatoes and drizzle with olive oil.

Bake in the oven for 15–20 minutes until the crust is golden and the tomatoes are soft. The tomatoes will have disintegrated slightly under the crust. Scatter with more parsley to serve.

Butternut Squash Soup with Parmesan Crostini

CALORIES PER SERVING: 185

Serves 4 | Preparation time: 40 minutes | Cooking time: 50 minutes

Creamy butternut squash is ideal for puréeing, and both the sharpness of the Parmesan and the crisp bite of the crostini set it off beautifully to produce a special soup. It also freezes well, so store some away for a cold night.

2 tbsp olive oil

1 large leek, trimmed and sliced thickly

1 celery stick, chopped

1 garlic clove chopped

1 tbsp chopped fresh sage

1 small red chile, halved and deseeded

12oz (350g) peeled, deseeded and diced (see note) butternut squash

4¼c (1 liter) vegetable stock

a pinch of cayenne pepper

salt and pepper

for the Parmesan crostini

4 thin slices day-old ciabatta or French bread

2 garlic cloves, peeled

extra virgin olive oil, for drizzling

1oz (25g) Parmesan cheese

Preheat the oven to 400°F/200°C. Heat the oil in a saucepan, add the leek, celery and garlic and fry gently for 10 minutes. Add the sage, chile and squash, and stir-fry for 5 minutes until the squash begins to color.

Pour in the stock, add the cayenne and bring to a boil. Cover and simmer for 35 minutes, then transfer to a food processor and blend until smooth. Return to the pan, adjust the seasoning with salt and pepper and heat through.

Meanwhile, make the crostini. Place the bread on a baking sheet and bake in the oven for 10 minutes. Rub each side with garlic, drizzle with a little oil and return to the oven for another 10 minutes or until the bread is crisp and golden.

Spoon the soup into warmed bowls, and top with the crostini. Grate the Parmesan over the top and drizzle on a little more oil. Serve at once.

Note: To give this prepared weight of squash you will need about 1lb (450g).

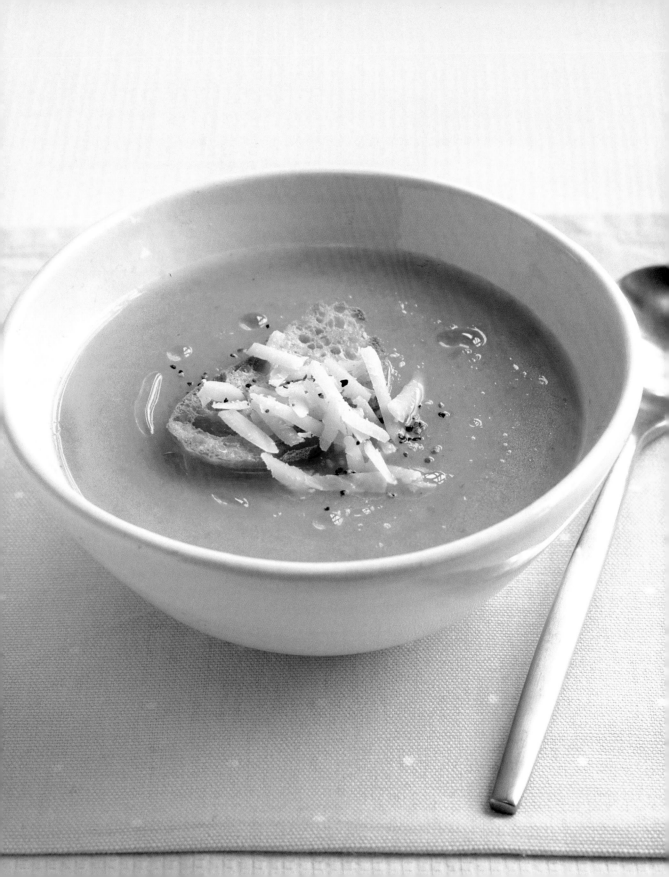

Lemon Chicken

CALORIES PER SERVING: 190

Serves 4 | Preparation time: 20 minutes, plus marinating time | Cooking time: 45 minutes

Corn-fed chicken pieces are marinated in lemon juice, chile and garlic, with a touch of honey. Ripe, juicy lemon halves are tucked in and around the joints to impart extra flavor during roasting.

1 x 3.5lb (.6 kg) corn-fed
    chicken, or 4 large
    chicken pieces
4 really ripe juicy
    lemons
8 garlic cloves
2 small red chiles,
    halved and
    deseeded
1 tbsp honey
4 tbsp chopped flat-leaf
    parsley
salt and pepper

Using a sharp knife and/or poultry shears, cut the whole chicken, if using, into 8 small or 4 large pieces. Place the chicken pieces, skin-side down, in a large shallow ovenproof baking dish.

Halve the lemons, squeeze the juice and pour into a small bowl; reserve the empty lemon halves.

Crush two of the garlic cloves and add to the lemon juice. Add the chiles and honey. Stir well, pour over the chicken and tuck in the lemon halves. Cover and leave to marinate for at least 2 hours, turning once or twice.

Preheat the oven to 400°F/200°C. Turn the chicken skin-side up. Halve the rest of the garlic cloves and scatter over the chicken. Roast in the oven for 45 minutes or until golden brown and tender. Stir in the parsley and season with salt and pepper, to taste. Serve hot, garnished with the roasted lemon halves.

Tomato and Peach Salad with Avocado Salsa

CALORIES PER SERVING: 195

Serves 4 | Preparation time: 15 minutes | Cooking time: 3 minutes

This is a really attractive platter—add a few chive flowers or decorative edible leaves if you have any growing close at hand.

1 large ripe beef steak
   tomato
2 large firm ripe
   peaches
chopped chives, to serve
cilantro sprigs, to serve
lime wedges, to serve

for the avocado salsa
½ small ripe avocado
2 spring onions,
   trimmed
1 small red chile
1 garlic clove, crushed
1½ tsp lime juice
1½ tsp chopped cilantro
1½ tsp extra virgin olive oil
salt and pepper

for the dressing
1 tbsp baker's sugar
1 tsp lemon juice
½ tsp Dijon mustard
2 tbsp extra virgin olive oil
salt and pepper

First prepare the avocado salsa. Peel and dice the avocado, and finely slice the spring onions. Halve, deseed and finely chop the chile. Mix these ingredients together in a bowl and stir in the garlic, lime juice, cilantro and oil. Season with salt and pepper, to taste, and set aside until required.

To prepare the dressing, dissolve the sugar in 3 tbsp (50ml) water in a small pan over low heat. Bring to a boil and simmer for 3 minutes. Remove from the heat, allow to cool, then stir in the lemon juice and mustard. Gradually whisk in the oil until emulsified and season with salt and pepper, to taste.

Thinly slice the tomato. Halve and slice the peaches and remove the pits. Scatter the tomato and peach slices on a large plate.

Spoon the avocado salsa on top and drizzle on the dressing. Sprinkle with chives and garnish with cilantro sprigs and lime wedges. Serve at once.

Note: Allow the salsa to stand while preparing the rest of the salad, but no longer or the avocado will discolor and spoil the appearance of the dish.

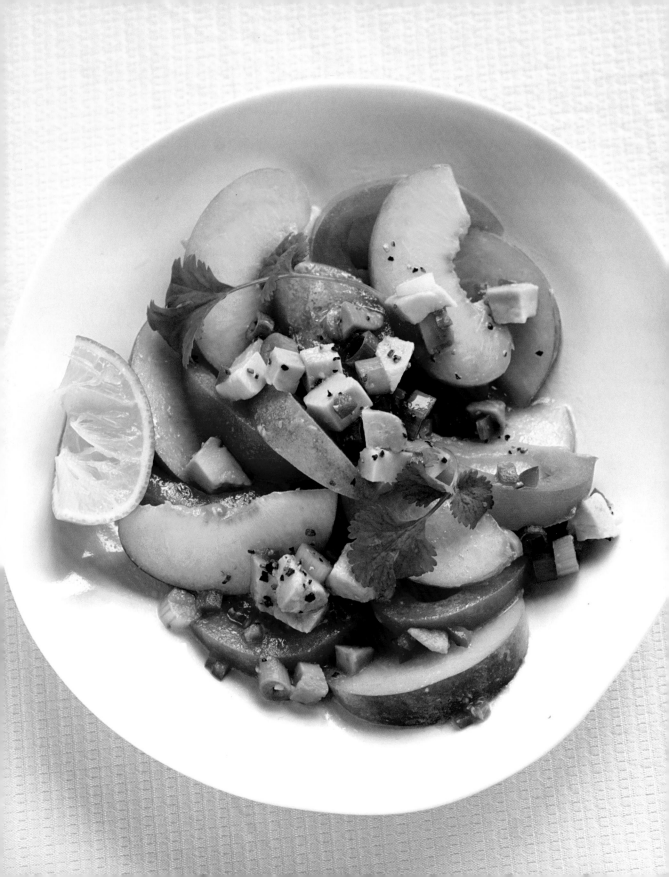

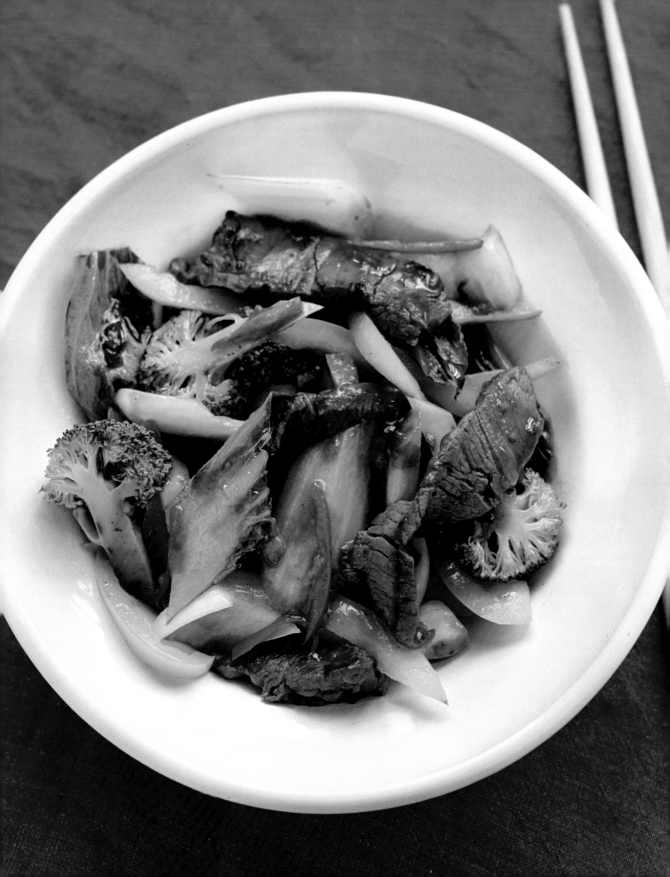

Chinese Beef

CALORIES PER SERVING: 200

Serves 4 │ Preparation time: 20 minutes, plus marinating time │ Cooking time: 15 minutes

Quickly cooked in very little oil, the natural flavors and textures of the vegetables in this dish are retained. Tender strips of beef are marinated in a rich sauce of black and yellow bean sauce.

12oz (350g) fillet steak
2 bunches of spring
    onions
2 orange peppers
1 red chile
8oz (225g) broccoli
6oz (175g) spinach (or
    bok choy)
1 tbsp chili oil

for the marinade
2 tbsp sherry vinegar
2 tbsp black bean sauce
2 tbsp yellow bean
    sauce
1in (2.5cm) piece fresh
    ginger root
1 tbsp dark soy sauce

First, prepare the marinade. Mix the sherry vinegar with the black and yellow bean sauces. Peel and crush the ginger and add to the mixture with the soy sauce.

Slice the fillet steak into thin strips, about 2in (5cm) long and ½in (1cm) wide. Stir into the marinade. Cover and leave to marinate in a cool place for at least 30 minutes or up to 12 hours in the fridge.

Trim the spring onions and cut into diagonal strips about 2in (5cm) long. Cut the peppers and chile in half, and remove and discard the seeds. Slice the peppers into thin strips; cut the chile into very fine strips. Cut the broccoli into small, even florets. Shred the spinach.

Drain the meat from the marinade, using a slotted spoon. Heat the oil in a large non-stick frying pan or wok over high heat, add the meat and cook for 3–4 minutes, stirring. Stir in the vegetables and cook for 3–4 minutes. Stir in the marinade and heat through for 3–4 minutes. Serve immediately.

Lime-Marinated Halibut
with Avocado and Red Onion Salsa

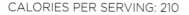

CALORIES PER SERVING: 210

Serves 4 | Preparation time: 10 minutes, plus marinating

This recipe is based on the famous South American dish ceviche—raw fish marinated in citrus juices. The acid from the fruit "cooks" the fish, but retains the texture, keeping it moist. Your fish must be very fresh.

20oz (575g) halibut
juice of 1 orange
juice of 5 limes

for the salsa
1 red pepper
1 red chile
1 small red onion
1 beef tomato
1 small avocado
4 tbsp chopped cilantro
2 tbsp chopped flat-leaf
    parsley
¼ tsp salt
pepper

Remove any skin and bones from the fish, and cut into bite-size pieces. Place in a bowl with the orange juice and lime juice. Turn the fish and make sure that it is all covered with citrus juice. Cover the bowl and leave to marinate in the refrigerator for at least 8 hours, or preferably overnight.

To make the salsa, halve the pepper, remove the core and seeds, then dice the flesh. Cut the chile in half lengthways, remove the seeds and chop very finely. Peel and dice the red onion. Mix all these ingredients together in a bowl.

Immerse the tomato in a small bowl of boiling water, leave for 30 seconds, then refresh in cold water. Peel away the skin. Cut the tomato into quarters, remove the seeds, then dice the flesh.

Cut the avocado in half, remove the pit and peel away the skin. Dice the flesh. Add to the onion mixture with the tomato, cilantro, parsley, salt and pepper, to taste. Mix together well. Serve the marinated fish on individual plates topped with a spoonful of salsa.

Note: If a smoother sauce is preferred, the salsa ingredients can be puréed in a blender or food processor.

Minted Lamb

CALORIES PER SERVING: 210

Serves 6 | Preparation time: 10 minutes, plus marinating time | Cooking time: 6 minutes

Extra-lean, wafer-thin lamb slices are flavored with a fresh-tasting minted yogurt marinade, then grilled to perfection.

1lb (450g) lean lamb
    slices, flattened
¼ red onion, finely
    sliced
40g baby spinach
12 cherry tomatoes,
    halved
1 tbsp mint leaves, to
    garnish

for the marinade
6 slightly heaped tbsp
    Greek-style yogurt
1 garlic clove, crushed
4 tbsp chopped mint
2 tbsp lemon juice
salt and pepper

For the marinade, mix the yogurt, crushed garlic, chopped mint and lemon juice together in a shallow non-metallic dish. Season with salt and pepper. Add the lamb and turn to coat evenly. Cover the dish and leave to marinate in a cool place for 2–3 hours.

Preheat the grill to high. Place the lamb on the grill rack in a single layer. Grill for 3 minutes on each side or until golden brown and cooked through, basting occasionally with the marinade.

Slice the lamb. Toss the red onion, spinach and tomatoes together, then divide among serving plates. Top with the lamb and mint leaves.

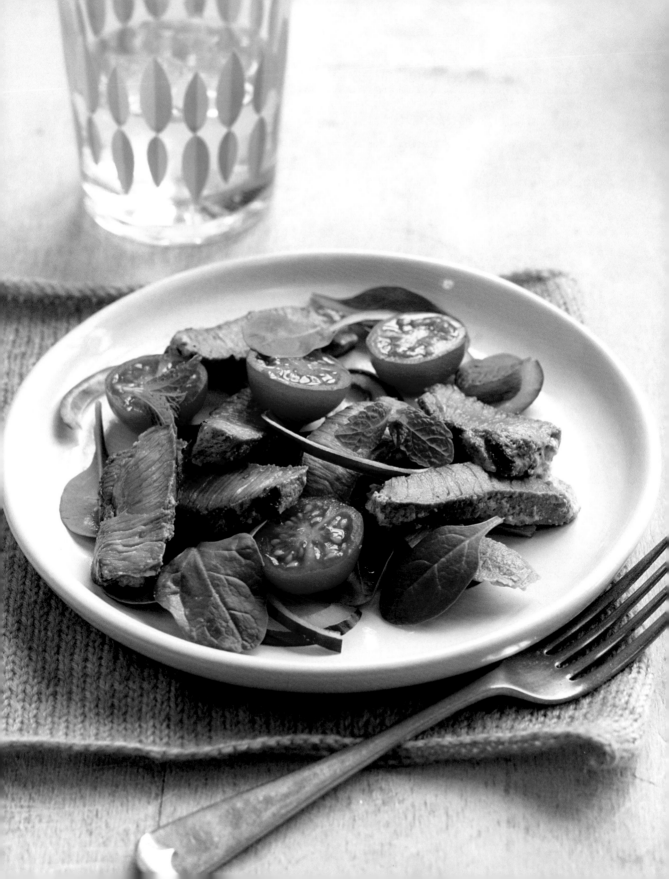

Vegetable Rice Noodles with Omelet Strips

CALORIES PER SERVING: 230

Serves 4 | Preparation time: 20 minutes | Cooking time: 10 minutes

Transparent noodles are tossed with stir-fried vegetables and topped with cilantro omelet shreds.

1in (2.5cm) piece fresh
    ginger root
6oz (175g) shiitake or
    button mushrooms
30g Chinese cabbage
1 red chile
¼lb (125g) rice noodles
1 tsp vegetable oil
1 tbsp peanut oil
4.5oz (125g) snow peas
2.5oz (75g) bean
    sprouts
2 tbsp dark soy sauce
2 tbsp dry sherry
1 tsp sugar

for the omelet
2 medium eggs
2 tbsp low-fat milk
3 tbsp chopped cilantro
1 tsp vegetable oil
salt and pepper

To make the omelet, whisk together the eggs, milk and cilantro. Season with salt and pepper.

Heat the oil in an omelet pan or small frying pan. Pour in the egg mixture and cook over high heat until it begins to set. As it sets around the edge, use an offset spatula to pull the set mixture toward the middle, letting the uncooked mixture run underneath. Cook until the egg is set all over.

Turn the omelet out onto a sheet of non-stick baking parchment and leave to cool. When cool, roll up and cut into thin slices.

Peel and shred the ginger. Thickly slice the mushrooms. Coarsely shred the Chinese cabbage. Slice the chile, removing the seeds if a milder flavor is preferred.

Cook the noodles according to the instructions on the package. Drain well and toss in a little vegetable oil.

Heat the peanut oil in a wok. Add the mushrooms and ginger and stir-fry over high heat for 2 minutes. Add the chile, snow peas, bean sprouts and shredded cabbage and stir-fry for 1 minute. Add the soy sauce, sherry and sugar and cook for 1 minute to heat through. Add the noodles to the pan and toss to mix, being careful not to crush them. (Don't worry if they won't mix properly).

Turn the vegetables and noodles into a warmed serving bowl and top with the omelet shreds.

Chicken with a Simple Vegetable Stew

CALORIES PER SERVING: 238

Serves 2 | Preparation time: 10 minutes | Cooking time: 25 minutes

This quick and comforting dish is perfect for midweek cooking. Celery root is very filling and has a lovely mild flavor.

2 x 4oz (125g) chicken
    breasts
3 tsp olive oil
zest of 1 lemon
1 rosemary sprig, leaves
    chopped
1c (250ml) hot chicken
    stock
1 shallot, sliced
½ celery root, chopped
2 carrots, chopped
4 stems broccolini
salt and pepper

Slash the chicken breasts a couple of times. Rub 1 teaspoon of the oil all over each piece of chicken. Then season with salt and pepper and rub in the lemon and rosemary. Heat a non-stick frying pan over a medium heat and fry the chicken for about 5 minutes on one side until golden.

Turn the chicken over and cook for 5 minutes on the other side. Add ⅓c (100ml) hot stock to the pan, cover and continue to cook over low heat for 15 minutes until cooked all the way through.

Meanwhile, heat the remaining teaspoon of olive oil in a pan and sauté the shallot for a minute or two until starting to turn golden. Add the celery root and carrots, stir to mix everything together and pour in the remaining stock. Cover and simmer for 10 minutes until the celery root is tender. Add the broccolini for the last 3 minutes of the cooking time. Season and serve, spooning the stock over the vegetables and the chicken juices over the chicken.

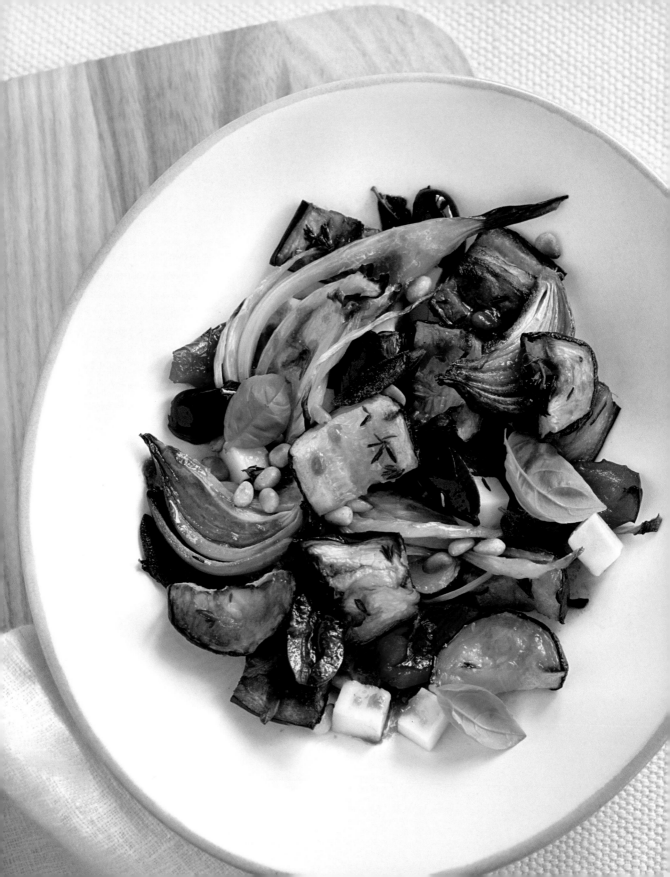

Warm Roasted Vegetable Salad

CALORIES PER SERVING: 240

Serves 4 | Preparation time: 20 minutes | Cooking time: 40 minutes

Port Salut melts beautifully and here it is tossed with warm roasted vegetables to impart a wonderfully creamy texture.

1 medium eggplant

1 medium zucchini

1 small red onion

½ fennel bulb, trimmed

1 red pepper

½ tbsp chopped thyme

½ tbsp chopped sage

2 tbsp olive oil, plus a
    little extra to drizzle

½ small head of garlic

2.25oz (64g) Port Salut
    or havarti cheese,
    diced

1 tbsp chopped basil

0.5oz (12g) pitted black
    olives

1½ tbsp (12g) pine nuts,
    toasted

salt and pepper

basil leaves, to garnish

for the dressing

1 tsp balsamic or sherry
    vinegar

2 tbsp extra virgin olive oil

Preheat the oven to 450°F/230°C. Cut the eggplant and zucchini into 1in (2.5cm) cubes. Layer in a large colander, sprinkling with a teaspoon of salt. Set aside for 30 minutes. Rinse the vegetables thoroughly to remove the salt and dry well with a paper towel.

Cut the onion into small wedges. Remove the tough outer layer and core from the fennel, then cut into small dice. Halve, core and deseed the pepper, then cut into 1in (2.5cm) squares.

Combine all of the vegetables in a large bowl. Add the thyme, sage and oil, toss well, then transfer to a roasting pan large enough to hold the vegetables in a single layer.

Stand the half garlic head on a small sheet of foil. Drizzle over a little oil, season with salt and pepper, and seal the foil to form a packet. Set the packet among the vegetables and roast for about 40 minutes, stirring the vegetables from time to time to ensure they brown evenly. Transfer the vegetables to a large bowl and stir in the cheese.

Unwrap the garlic and scoop out the flesh into a bowl. Add the dressing ingredients, season with salt and pepper, and whisk to combine.

Pour the garlic dressing over the vegetables. Add the chopped basil, olives and pine nuts and toss lightly. Serve immediately, garnished with basil leaves.

Grilled Tomato and Mozzarella Salad

CALORIES PER SERVING: 240

Serves 4 | Preparation time: 10 minutes | Cooking time: 10 minutes

This hot salad can be prepared ahead, chilled, then grilled just before serving. Make sure you use tomatoes that are ripe and have plenty of flavor.

6oz (175g) eggplant

3 tbsp olive oil

1lb (450g) ripe
   tomatoes

5.25oz (150g)
   mozzarella cheese

4 tbsp torn basil leaves

finely grated zest of 1 lemon

1 tsp lemon juice

salt and pepper

basil leaves, to garnish

Preheat the grill to medium. Cut the eggplant into thin slices. Brush very lightly with some of the oil and place on the grill rack. Grill the eggplant slices on both sides until they are crisp and golden brown; do not let them turn too dark at this stage.

Thinly slice the tomatoes. Cut the mozzarella cheese into thin slices.

In a bowl, whisk together the remaining oil, torn basil, lemon zest and juice. Season with salt and pepper.

Arrange the tomato, eggplant and mozzarella slices, overlapping in a single layer, in a large shallow ovenproof dish. Spoon the dressing evenly over the top.

Place under a hot broiler for 3–4 minutes or until the mozzarella begins to melt.

Sprinkle with salt and pepper and garnish with basil leaves. Serve immediately.

Fruit and Prawn Salad with Chili Dressing

CALORIES PER SERVING: 240

Serves 4 | Preparation time: 15 minutes | Cooking time: 2 minutes

This Indonesian salad is an unusual combination of exotic fruits and cooked prawns. Accompanied by a hot and sour dressing, it is bursting with a whole range of exciting flavors.

1 firm ripe papaya
1 pink grapefruit
1 small firm ripe mango
1 large firm ripe banana
12 large cooked prawns
    in shells
orange zest, to garnish

for the dressing
1½ tbsp lemon juice
1 tbsp rice wine vinegar
1 tbsp baker's sugar
1 tsp dark soy sauce
¼ tsp crushed red chiles
2 tbsp peanut oil
pinch of salt

First make the dressing. Place the lemon juice, vinegar, sugar, soy sauce and chiles in a small saucepan and heat gently to dissolve the sugar. Remove from the heat and whisk in the oil and salt. Leave to cool.

Prepare the fruits. Peel and halve the papaya, then scoop out the seeds and thinly slice the flesh. Peel the grapefruit, removing all of the white pith, and cut out the segments between the membranes. Peel the mango, cut the flesh away from the stone, then cut into slices. Peel and slice the banana.

Arrange the fruits on a large serving platter and spoon over the dressing. Peel the prawns, leaving on the tail end shells. Arrange on top of the salad and garnish with orange zest. Serve immediately.

Herb Gnocchi with Grilled Tomato Sauce

CALORIES PER SERVING: 245

Serves 4 | Preparation time: 25 minutes | Cooking time: 30 minutes

Gnocchi are very filling, so you only need a small portion. Here they are served with a grilled tomato sauce, which has a lovely smoky flavor. Use a combination of red and yellow cherry tomatoes if possible, as this looks really stunning.

1lb (450g) russet
   potatoes, peeled
   and halved
1 medium egg
1 tsp salt
1 tbsp finely chopped
   rosemary
½c less 1 tbsp (60g)
   all-purpose flour
freshly grated Parmesan
   cheese, to serve
rosemary sprigs, to
   garnish

for the sauce
1lb (450g) mixed red
   and yellow cherry
   tomatoes
2 garlic cloves, sliced
1 tsp grated lemon zest
1 tbsp chopped thyme
1 tbsp chopped basil
2 tbsp olive oil
a pinch of sugar
salt and pepper

Cook the potatoes in lightly salted boiling water for 15-20 minutes until cooked; drain well and return to the pan. Set over a gentle heat to dry the potatoes out and leave to cool slightly.

Bring a large pan of water to a steady simmer. Mash the potatoes smoothly, then work in the egg, salt, rosemary and enough flour to form a soft dough. Add a little more flour if the mixture is too sticky. Transfer to a piping bag fitted with a large plain nozzle.

Meanwhile make the sauce. Preheat the grill to high. Halve the tomatoes and place in an ovenproof dish. Add the garlic, lemon zest, herbs, oil and seasoning and toss together. Sprinkle over the sugar and grill for 10 minutes until the tomatoes are charred and tender.

While the tomatoes are grilling, cook the gnocchi in batches. Pipe about six 2in (5cm) lengths directly into the boiling water, using a sharp knife to cut them off at the nozzle. Cook for 3-4 minutes, until the gnocchi float to the surface.

Remove with a slotted spoon, drain on paper towels and transfer to a large warmed bowl. Toss with a little olive oil and keep warm in the oven while cooking the remaining potato mixture.

Toss the cooked gnocchi with the grilled tomato sauce. Serve immediately, dusted with a little freshly grated Parmesan and garnished with rosemary.

Root Vegetable and Lentil Casserole

CALORIES PER SERVING: 260

Serves 6 | Preparation time: 20 minutes | Cooking time: 1 hour

This spicy combination of mixed root vegetables and assorted lentils makes a hearty, filling supper dish.

1 tsp cumin seeds
1 tbsp coriander seeds
1 tsp mustard seeds
1oz (25g) fresh ginger
    root
3 tbsp olive oil
3 onions, sliced
1lb (450g) carrots,
    chopped
12oz (350g) leeks,
    trimmed and sliced
12oz (350g) daikon
    radish, peeled and
    roughly chopped
1lb (450g) button
    mushrooms, halved
2 garlic cloves, crushed
¼ tsp ground turmeric
6oz (175g) split red
    lentils
2oz (50g) brown or
    green lentils
2 tbsp chopped cilantro
    leaves
salt and pepper
parsley sprigs, to
    garnish

Preheat the oven to 350°F/180°C. Crush the cumin, coriander and mustard seeds in a mortar with a pestle. Peel and grate or finely chop the ginger.

Heat the oil in a large ovenproof Dutch oven. Add the onions, carrots, leeks and daikon, and fry for 2–3 minutes, stirring constantly. Add the mushrooms, garlic, ginger, turmeric and crushed spices, and fry for another 2–3 minutes, stirring.

Rinse the lentils in a colander under cold running water, then drain. Stir the lentils into the pan with 3c (750ml) boiling water. Season with salt and pepper and return to a boil. Cover and cook in the oven for about 45 minutes or until the vegetables and lentils are tender. Stir in the cilantro and adjust the seasoning before serving, garnished with parsley.

Roasted Chicken with a Deviled Sauce

CALORIES PER SERVING: 270

Serves 6 │ Preparation time: 20 minutes │ Cooking time: 1 hour 45 minutes

When roasts were the mainstay of British cooking, "deviling"—using a hot sauce—was a popular way of reviving leftovers. Here, the idea is put to better use. A hot, tangy base is used for glazing a large chicken during roasting; it also forms the basis of a delicious sauce. For a more fiery sauce, add a finely chopped chile to the deviled mixture before basting.

1 x 5lb (2.3kg) chicken
1 large onion
3 garlic cloves
⅓c (90ml) crème
    fraîche
leafy herbs (e.g., basil,
    lovage or lemon
    balm), to garnish

for the deviled sauce
2 tbsp mango chutney
1½ tbsp (25g) butter
2 tbsp Worcestershire
    sauce
2 tbsp grainy mustard
1 tsp paprika
3 tbsp freshly squeezed
    orange juice
1lb (450g) tomatoes
salt and pepper

Preheat the oven to 375°F/190°C. To make the deviled sauce, chop any large pieces in the chutney. Melt the butter. Mix together the butter, chutney, Worcestershire sauce, mustard, paprika, orange juice and seasoning.

Peel and chop the onion and garlic; place in the cavity of the chicken, then place the chicken in a roasting pan. Baste the skin all over with the deviled sauce. Roast in the oven, basting frequently with the sauce for 1 hour and 45 minutes, or until the juices run clear when the thickest part of the thigh is pierced with a skewer. At the end of the cooking time the chicken should be slightly charred, but cover with foil toward the end of cooking if it starts to darken too much.

Meanwhile, place the tomatoes in a bowl and cover with boiling water. Leave for 30 seconds, then drain and peel the skins. Scoop out the seeds and roughly chop the tomatoes.

Transfer the chicken to a warmed serving platter and keep warm. Skim off the fat from the juices in the roasting pan, then stir in the tomatoes and any remaining deviled sauce. Transfer the sauce to a food processor or blender and process briefly until the mixture is pulpy but retaining a little texture. Return to the pan and heat through, seasoning with salt and pepper to taste.

Meanwhile warm the crème fraîche in a small saucepan. Garnish the chicken with plenty of herbs and serve with the deviled sauce and crème fraîche.

Chicken with Herby Nut Stuffing

CALORIES PER SERVING: 307

Serves 4 │ Preparation time: 15 minutes │ Cooking time: 1 hour

This is a deconstructed roasted chicken with stuffing. The chicken is kept juicy by being cooked in stock, while the stuffing has a satisfying crunch.

4 x 4.5oz (125g) skinless
  chicken breasts
1 tsp dried rosemary or
  thyme
1 tsp olive oil
1¼c (300ml) hot
  chicken stock
salt and pepper

for the stuffing
1 tbsp (15g) butter
1 tsp olive oil
1 small onion, finely
  chopped
1 large zucchini, finely
  chopped
1 celery stick, finely
  chopped
½ apple, grated
0.5oz (10g) almonds,
  toasted and chopped
0.5oz (10g) raisins,
  chopped
3.5oz (100g) day-old
  whole wheat bread,
  processed into
  breadcrumbs
zest of ½ lemon
1 tsp dried rosemary or
  thyme
1 medium egg, beaten

Slash the chicken all over and season well with the dried herbs, salt and pepper, and rub in the oil. Set aside.

Make the stuffing. Heat the butter and oil in a pan and add the onion, zucchini and celery. Sauté over low heat for 10–15 minutes until the onion has softened and the vegetables start to caramelize. Tip into a bowl to cool.

Once cool, add the remaining stuffing ingredients. Mix well, then spoon into a small ovenproof dish or loaf tin. Cover with foil.

Preheat the oven to 375°F/190°C. Line a small loaf pan or ovenproof dish with parchment paper. Heat a non-stick frying pan and pan-fry the chicken for 2–3 minutes on each side until golden. Transfer to the prepared loaf pan or ovenproof dish and pour over the stock. Cover with foil.

Cook the chicken and stuffing in the oven for 45–50 minutes until the chicken is cooked through and the stuffing is golden and slightly crisp on top. Serve each chicken breast with a piece of stuffing and the stock spooned over the top.

Fava Bean and Pecorino Salad

CALORIES PER SERVING: 310

Serves 4 │ Preparation time: 30 minutes │ Cooking time: 1 minute

You can use frozen fava beans for this dish with good effect, but it is worth waiting until your own local fava beans are harvested to truly appreciate this salad.

1lb (450g) shelled fava beans

4 heads of red chicory, trimmed

2oz (50g) hard pecorino cheese

½ small red onion

1oz (25g) hazelnuts, toasted

salt

for the dressing

2 tsp raspberry vinegar

½ tsp honey

4 tbsp hazelnut oil

salt and pepper

Bring a large pan of lightly salted water to a rolling boil, add the fava beans, return to a boil and cook for 1 minute. Drain and immediately refresh under cold water. Drain and pat dry. Carefully remove and discard the tough outer skins by pinching one end of the skin to release the inner bean, then place the fava beans in a large bowl.

Separate the chicory into leaves and add to the beans. Using a vegetable peeler, finely pare the cheese. Thinly slice the onion. Roughly chop the hazelnuts.

To make the dressing, place the vinegar, honey and seasoning in a small jug and gradually whisk in the oil until blended. Pour half of the dressing over the beans and chicory and toss until well coated.

Arrange the beans and chicory on individual serving plates, top with the cheese, onion and nuts and drizzle the remaining dressing on top. Serve at once.

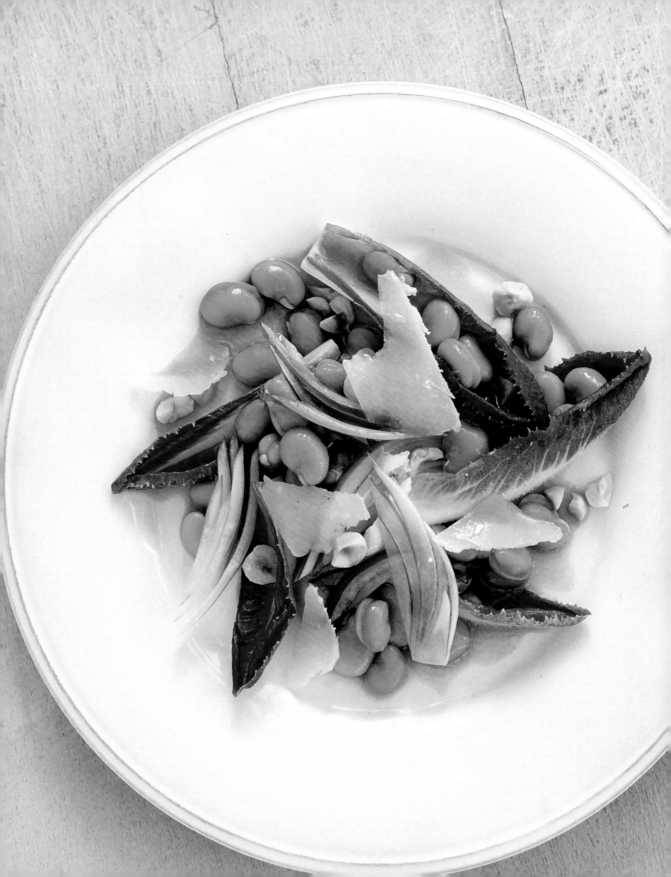

Grilled Jumbo Prawns with a Spicy Tomato and Pepper Sauce

CALORIES PER SERVING: 315

Serves 4 | Preparation time: 10 minutes | Cooking time: 40 minutes

This recipe is based on a classic Spanish romesco sauce, which can be served with almost any fish, hot or cold. Choose prawns of equal sizes.

24 raw jumbo prawns in shell
3 tbsp olive oil
flat-leaf parsley, to garnish

for the sauce
4 garlic cloves
2 ripe plum tomatoes
4 tbsp olive oil
1 onion, chopped
1 pimento pepper in oil, drained and chopped
½ tsp dried chili flakes
5 tbsp fish stock
2 tbsp white wine
10 blanched almonds
1 tbsp red wine vinegar
salt

To make the sauce, chop the garlic, setting aside one of the chopped cloves.

Immerse the tomatoes in a bowl of boiling water for 30 seconds, then refresh in cold water. Drain, then peel away the skins. Roughly chop the tomato flesh.

Heat 2 tablespoons of the oil in a pan, add the onion and garlic, and cook gently until softened. Add the chopped tomatoes and pimento, together with the chili flakes, stock and wine. Cover and simmer for 30 minutes.

Preheat the grill to medium and spread the almonds on a baking sheet. Toast the almonds under the grill until golden; alternatively toast them in a pan. Transfer to a food processor or blender and grind coarsely. Add the remaining oil, the vinegar, reserved garlic and salt to taste. Purée until evenly combined. Add the tomato sauce and blend until smooth.

Remove the heads from the prawns and, using a sharp knife, slit each one down the back and remove the black intestinal vein. Rinse in cold water, and dry on paper towels.

Preheat the grill. Toss the prawns in the oil, then spread out in the grill pan in an even layer. Grill for about 2–3 minutes on each side, until the shells have turned pink. Arrange on a serving platter, garnish with parsley and serve with the sauce.

Chicken with Tomato and Orange Sauce

CALORIES PER SERVING: 315

Serves 4 | Preparation time: 20 minutes | Cooking time: 35–40 minutes

These chicken breasts are filled with a light, fresh mixture of ricotta cheese, herbs and garlic, and served with a delicate sauce of fresh tomatoes simmered with a little orange.

6oz (175g) ricotta
    cheese
4 tbsp chopped fresh
    mixed herbs (e.g.,
    oregano, thyme,
    parsley and chives)
2 garlic cloves, crushed
4 x 5oz (150g) skinless
    chicken breast fillets
4 slices of prosciutto
salt and pepper
leafy herbs (e.g., basil,
    or lemon balm), to
    garnish
orange wedges, to
    serve

for the sauce
12oz (350g) plum
    tomatoes
2 shallots, finely
    chopped
zest and juice of
    1 orange
1 garlic clove, crushed
1 tbsp orange
    marmalade
salt and pepper

Preheat the oven to 400°F/200°C. Place the ricotta cheese in a bowl and break up with a wooden spoon. Stir in the chopped herbs, garlic and seasoning.

Cut a 2in (5cm) pocket along one side of each chicken breast. Divide the filling into 4 portions and ease a portion into each pocket. Pull the chicken flesh together to encase the filling.

Wrap a slice of prosciutto around each chicken breast: lay the prosciutto over the breast, then fold the ends under to enclose and help seal in the filling.

Place the chicken breasts in an ovenproof dish, cover with foil and cook in the oven for 35–40 minutes.

Meanwhile, make the sauce. Place the tomatoes in a large bowl, pour over enough boiling water to cover and leave for 30 seconds. Lift from the bowl and remove the skins. Roughly chop the tomato flesh.

Peel and finely chop the shallots. Put the orange zest and 2 tablespoons of the juice into a large pan. Stir in the chopped tomatoes, garlic and seasoning, cover and place over medium heat to sweat for a few minutes. Stir in the marmalade. Bring to a boil, then simmer for about 20 minutes, until the mixture is of a spooning consistency.

Place the chicken breasts on warmed serving plates, spoon over the sauce, garnish with herbs and serve with orange wedges.

Roasted Vegetable Omelet

CALORIES PER SERVING: 320

Serves 2 | Preparation time: 5 minutes | Cooking time: 30–40 minutes

Omelets are very versatile and can be filled with endless combinations of flavors. This is a very filling, simple supper.

1 onion, peeled and cut into 6 wedges
10oz (300g) peeled butternut squash, cut into bite-size chunks
½ red pepper
2 tsp olive oil
4 broccoli florets
4 medium eggs
0.5oz (10g) Parmesan cheese, grated
salt and pepper

Preheat the oven to 400°F/200°C.

Arrange the onion, squash and pepper in a roasting pan. Whisk together 1 tablespoon of cold water and 1 teaspoon of the oil and drizzle over the vegetables. Season well and toss together. Roast in the oven for 30–40 minutes until the vegetables are tender.

Blanch the broccoli in a pan of boiling water until just tender, then drain.

Preheat the broiler to high. Beat the eggs in a bowl and season well. Heat the remaining olive oil in a medium non-stick ovenproof frying pan. Arrange the vegetables in the pan then pour the beaten eggs over the top.

Use a wooden spoon to draw the egg away from the sides of the pan, allowing some of the uncooked egg to run into the holes. Continue to do this for a few minutes until the egg looks almost cooked. Scatter the cheese on top and place under the broiler until the egg is just cooked.

Stir-Fried Beef with Noodles and Chili

CALORIES PER SERVING: 325

Serves 4 | Preparation time: 20 minutes | Cooking time: 15 minutes

For this quick noodle dish, minced beef is stir-fried with Indian curry paste, garlic, ginger and spices, then tossed with noodles and vegetables.

4.5oz (125g) dried egg
   noodles
3 tbsp vegetable oil
1 tbsp dark soy sauce
1 small onion, finely
   chopped
2 garlic cloves, finely
   chopped
1in (2.5cm) piece fresh
   ginger root
4 Kaffir lime leaves,
   shredded
8oz (225g) lean minced
   beef
2 tbsp Indian medium
   curry paste
1 tsp ground turmeric
½ tsp paprika
¼ tsp chili powder
1 red pepper, deseeded
   and sliced
4.5oz (125g) green
   beans, halved
cilantro leaves, to
   garnish

for the sauce
2 tbsp tamarind paste
1 tbsp Thai fish sauce
2 tsp sugar
⅓c (90ml) beef stock

Cook the noodles according to the packet instructions, drain well and pat dry.

Meanwhile prepare the sauce. Place the tamarind paste in a bowl and whisk in the remaining ingredients until smooth. Set aside.

Heat 1 tablespoon of the oil in a wok or large frying pan, add the noodles and soy sauce, and stir-fry for 30 seconds. Remove from the pan and set aside.

Add the remaining oil to the pan. Add the onion and garlic, then grate in the ginger and scatter over the lime leaves. Fry, stirring, for 5 minutes. Add the beef, curry paste and spices and stir-fry for 3 minutes.

Add the red pepper and beans, and stir-fry for 3 minutes. Mix in the sauce and simmer for another 3 minutes. Carefully stir in the noodles and heat through for 2 minutes. Transfer to a warmed serving dish and garnish with the cilantro.

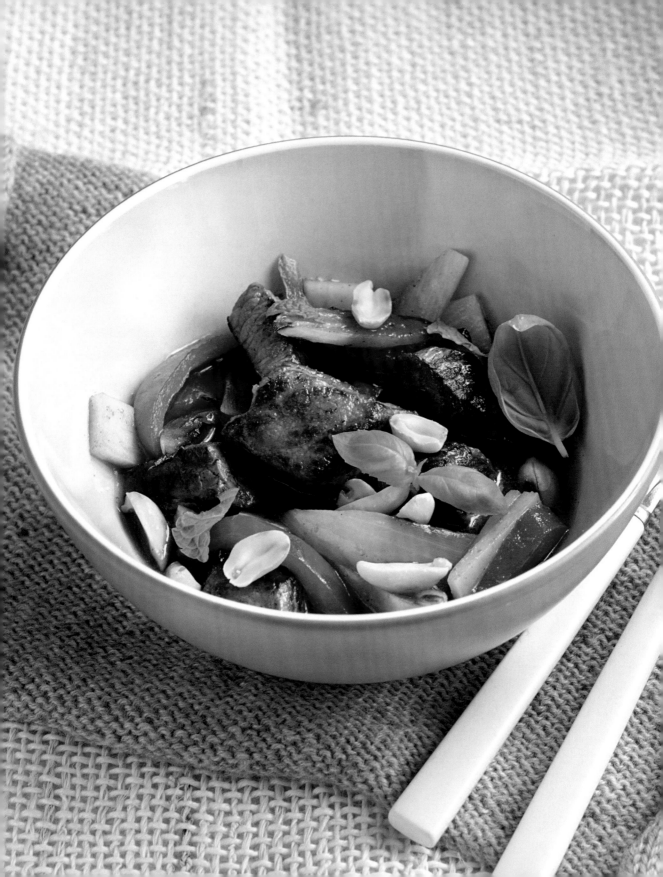

Lamb and Bamboo Shoot Red Curry

CALORIES PER SERVING: 325

Serves 4 | Preparation time: 30 minutes | Cooking time: 45 minutes

A fiery and satisfying meaty dish. The peanuts provide a wonderful crunch, contrasting with the juicy lamb.

1lb (450g) lean lamb
2 tbsp vegetable oil
1 large onion, cut into
  wedges
2 garlic cloves, finely
  chopped
2 tbsp Thai red curry
  paste
⅔c (150ml) lamb or
  beef stock
2 tbsp Thai fish sauce
2 tsp soft brown sugar
1 x 7oz (200g) can
  bamboo shoots,
  drained
1 red pepper, deseeded
2 tbsp chopped mint
1 tbsp chopped basil
1oz (25g) raw peanuts,
  toasted
basil leaves, to garnish

Cut the lamb into 1in (3cm) cubes. Heat the oil in a wok or large frying pan, add the onion and garlic, and fry over medium heat for 5 minutes.

Add the lamb together with the curry paste and stir-fry for 5 minutes. Add the stock, fish sauce and sugar. Bring to a boil, lower the heat, cover and simmer gently for 20 minutes.

Meanwhile, slice the bamboo shoots and red pepper. Stir into the curry with the herbs and cook, uncovered, for another 10 minutes. Stir in the peanuts and serve at once, garnished with basil leaves.

Turkey Melt

CALORIES PER SERVING: 332

Serves 2 | Preparation time: 10 minutes | Cooking time: 10 minutes

This chunky hot sandwich won't feel like it is low-calorie at all. It's a thoroughly satisfying, speedy and very flavorful supper.

2 x 4.5oz (125g) turkey
  breast fillets
2 tsp olive oil
1 tbsp apple chutney
1oz (20g) reduced-fat
  cheddar cheese
0.5oz (10g) whole
  wheat breadcrumbs
2 thin slices of
  sourdough bread
2 tomatoes, sliced
2oz (50g) salad greens
1 tsp balsamic vinegar
salt and pepper

Preheat the broiler to high. Season the turkey fillets with salt and pepper. Heat 1 teaspoon of the oil in a pan and fry the turkey for 2 minutes on each side, until cooked all the way through. Spread half a tablespoon of chutney over each piece.

Transfer to a baking sheet, sprinkle with the cheese and breadcrumbs and broil until golden.

Toast the slices of sourdough. Lay slices of tomato on top of each piece, top with the turkey and serve with the salad greens, tossed in the remaining teaspoon of oil and the balsamic vinegar.

Asparagus, Fava Bean and Parmesan Frittata

CALORIES PER SERVING: 350

Serves 4 | Preparation time: 35 minutes | Cooking time: 15–20 minutes

A pretty green frittata, full of fresh, clean flavors. You can use frozen fava beans for this dish—just make sure they are defrosted first.

6oz (175g) small
    fingerling potatoes
8oz (225g) asparagus
8oz (225g) shelled fava
    beans
6 medium eggs
2oz (50g) freshly grated
    Parmesan cheese
3 tbsp chopped mixed
    fresh herbs (e.g.,
    parsley, oregano and
    thyme)
3 tbsp (45g) butter
salt and pepper

Cook the potatoes in boiling salted water for 15–20 minutes until tender. Allow to cool, then slice thickly.

Meanwhile, trim the asparagus, removing any woody parts of the stems. Steam for 12 minutes until tender, then plunge into cold water to set the color and cool completely.

Slip the fava beans out of their waxy skins. Drain the asparagus, pat dry, then cut into short lengths. Mix with the fava beans.

Put the eggs in a bowl with a good pinch of salt, plenty of pepper and half of the Parmesan. Beat thoroughly until evenly blended, then stir in the asparagus, fava beans and chopped herbs.

Melt 2½ tbsp (40g) of the butter in a 10in (25cm) non-stick heavy-based frying pan. When foaming, pour in the egg mixture. Turn down the heat to as low as possible. Cook for about 15 minutes, until the frittata is set and the top is still a little runny.

Preheat the broiler to medium. Scatter the cooked sliced potato over the frittata and sprinkle with the remaining Parmesan. Dot with the rest of the butter.

Place under the hot broiler to brown the cheese lightly and just set the top; don't allow it to brown too much or it will dry out. Slide the frittata on to a warmed dish and cut into wedges to serve.

Chicken Breasts with Spinach and Ricotta

CALORIES PER SERVING: 360

Serves 4 | Preparation time: 30 minutes | Cooking time: 30–40 minutes

A popular recipe given a low-cal twist. The ricotta makes this an especially light but creamy option and the spinach adds a lovely flash of color.

2oz (50g) baby spinach

3.5oz (100g) ricotta cheese

1oz (20g) freshly grated Parmesan cheese

freshly grated nutmeg

4 x 5.25oz (150g) boneless, skinless chicken breasts

4 slices smoked pancetta

4 rosemary sprigs

⅔c (150ml) dry white wine

1¼c (300ml) hot chicken stock

2 tbsp (30g) butter, chilled and diced

9oz (250g) asparagus spears

salt and pepper

Preheat the oven to 400°F/200°C. Wilt the spinach in a pan and squeeze out any excess water, then roughly chop and place in a bowl. Add the ricotta, Parmesan and plenty of nutmeg, salt and pepper. Mix together well.

Using a sharp knife, make a deep horizontal slit in each chicken breast through the thicker side, to make a pocket. Spoon the filling evenly into the chicken pockets.

Wrap a slice of pancetta around each chicken breast, tucking a rosemary sprig into each. Secure with a toothpick, if necessary.

Lay the chicken breasts in a wide shallow pan or ovenproof casserole and pour in the wine and stock. Cook in the oven for 30–40 minutes until cooked through. Remove the chicken breasts with a slotted spoon and keep warm.

Bring the liquid to a boil. Simmer rapidly until reduced by half. Remove from the heat and whisk in the cubed butter, to enrich the sauce and give it a shine. Taste and adjust the seasoning. Steam the asparagus until tender.

Serve the chicken breasts on a plate with some asparagus alongside and a little sauce spooned over the top.

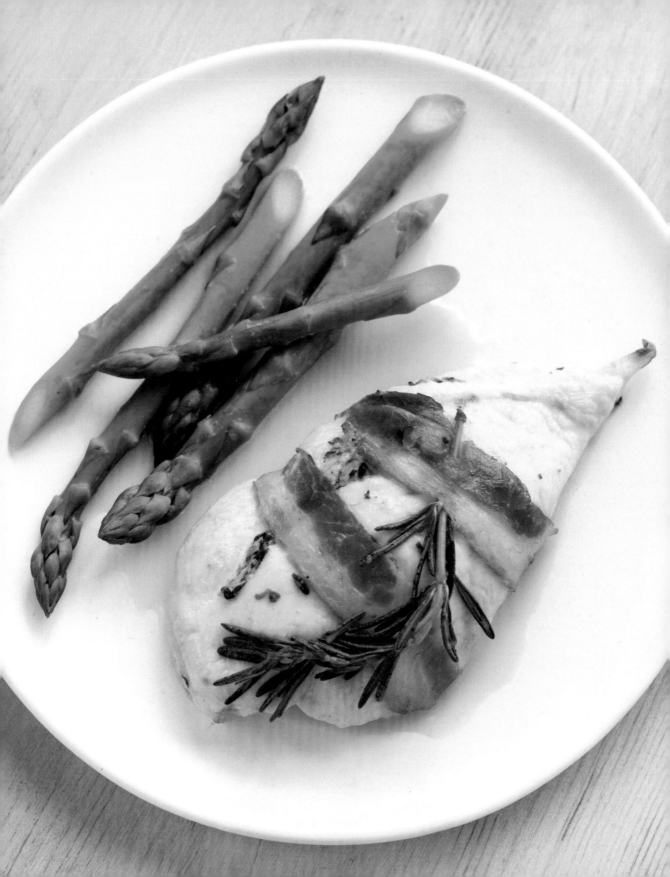

Braised Monkfish Wrapped in Prosciutto with French Green Lentils

CALORIES PER SERVING: 370

Serves 6 | Preparation time: 15 minutes, plus marinating | Cooking time: 40 minutes

Monkfish is a firm-fleshed fish, which can withstand cooking methods that are more suited to meat. Here the fish is wrapped in delicate thin slices of prosciutto, pan-fried until golden, and then gently braised on a bed of green lentils.

2lb (1kg) monkfish tail

1 small lemon

1 tbsp chopped fresh marjoram

6 thin slices of prosciutto

1 small onion

1 carrot

1 celery stick

1 garlic clove

3 tbsp olive oil

12oz (350g) French green lentils

⅔c (150ml) red wine

2 tomatoes, deseeded and diced

2oz (50g) spinach

salt and pepper

Fillet the monkfish by cutting down either side of the central bone. Peel the lemon, removing all the white pith, then cut into thin slices. Lay the fish cut-side up on a cutting board and sprinkle with the marjoram. Season with salt and pepper. Lay the lemon slices over one piece of fish, then sandwich together with the other half.

Wrap the fish in the prosciutto, making sure that it is completely covered. Tie at 2in (5cm) intervals with fine string. Cover and leave in a cool place for 1–2 hours.

Finely dice the onion, carrot and celery. Finely chop the garlic. Heat 2 tablespoons of the olive oil in a saucepan, add the garlic and vegetables, and cook, stirring, for about 8 minutes, until golden. Stir in the lentils and wine and add sufficient water to cover. Bring to a boil and cook for 10 minutes.

Heat the remaining oil in a large frying pan. Add the wrapped monkfish and fry, turning, until the prosciutto is browned all over. Carefully remove the wrapped fish and transfer the lentils and vegetables to the frying pan. Replace the fish on top, burying it into the lentils slightly. Cover the pan and cook over medium-low heat for 20 minutes, until the lentils are cooked and the juices from the fish run clear.

Quickly stir the tomatoes and spinach through the lentils. Serve the fish on a bed of lentils.

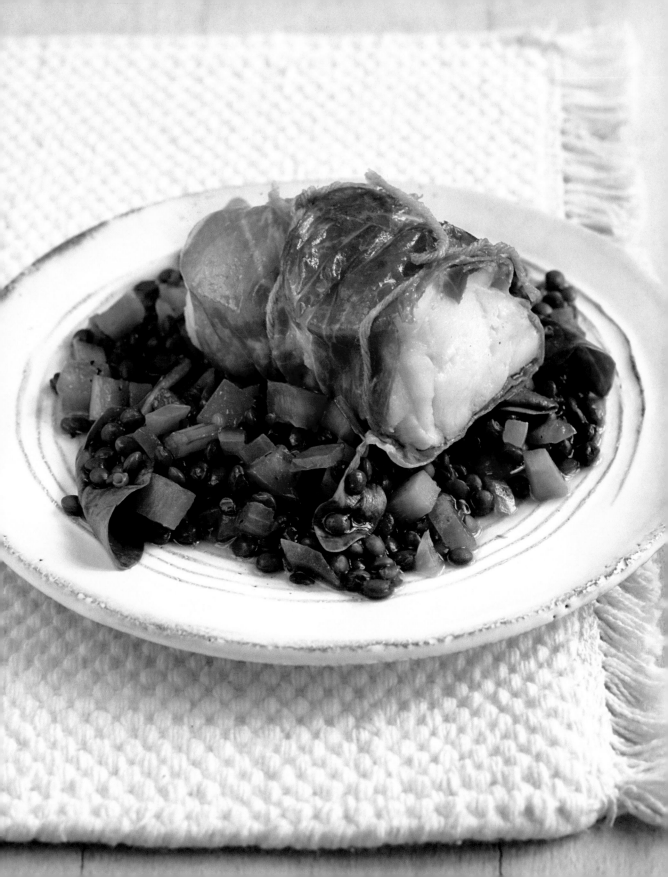

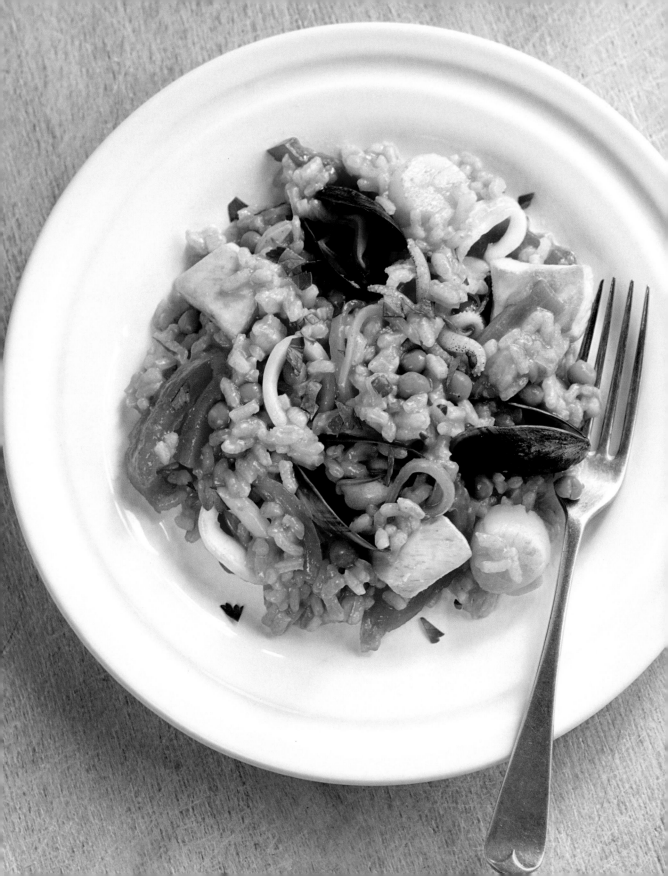

snacks and drinks

Koftas

CALORIES PER KOFTA: 40

Makes 24 | Preparation time: 20 minutes | Cooking time: 10 minutes

These make a fantastic snack and can be made well in advance, frozen and reheated straight from the freezer.

1 small onion, quartered
1 garlic clove, peeled
1in (2.5cm) piece fresh
    ginger root, halved
1 tsp ground cumin
1 tsp ground coriander
3 tbsp ghee or
    vegetable oil
1lb (450g) minced beef
3 tbsp chopped cilantro
1 medium egg
salt and pepper

Put the onion, garlic and ginger in a blender or food processor and work until finely chopped. Add the spices and process until evenly mixed.

Heat 1 tablespoon of the ghee or oil in a frying pan and add the onion paste. Cook over medium heat for 2–3 minutes, stirring all the time. Remove from the heat and allow to cool.

Put the minced beef in a bowl and break it up with a fork. Add the chopped cilantro and season with salt and pepper. Add the cooled onion paste and mix thoroughly until evenly incorporated. Add just enough beaten egg to bind; don't add too much or the mixture will be too sticky to shape.

Using lightly floured hands, shape the spiced beef mixture into 24 small balls.

Heat the remaining ghee or oil in the frying pan and add the koftas (see note). Cook for about 5 minutes or until browned on all sides and cooked through, shaking the pan as they cook to ensure they brown evenly. Drain the koftas on paper towels and serve hot.

Note: If your frying pan is small, you may need to cook the koftas in a couple of batches.

Spiced Ladyfingers

CALORIES PER LADYFINGER: 50

Makes 18 | Preparation time: 12 minutes | Cooking time: 15 minutes

Crisp and light with a slightly chewy center, these simple ladyfingers have an almost meringue-like texture. The deliciously spicy aftertaste is accentuated by the sprinkling of black pepper, although this can be omitted for a more conventional ladyfinger. These ladyfingers cannot be frozen but if stored in an airtight jar will last for up to a week.

1 medium egg white
2 tsp cornflour
½ tsp ground cinnamon
½ tsp ground ginger
⅔c (125g) baker's sugar
2.5oz (75g) ground
    almonds
black pepper and extra
    spices, for sprinkling

Preheat the oven to 350°F/180°C. Line a large baking sheet with parchment paper.

Whisk the egg white in a bowl until stiff, but not dry. Sift in the cornflour and spices. Add the sugar and ground almonds and gently stir the ingredients together to form a light, sticky paste.

Place the mixture in a large piping bag, fitted with a ½in (1cm) plain nozzle. Pipe 2¾in (7cm) finger lengths on to the baking sheet, spacing them slightly apart. Sprinkle with pepper and a little extra spices and bake for 12 minutes or until crisp and golden. Transfer to a wire rack to cool.

Note: If you don't have a suitable piping nozzle, spoon the mixture onto the lined baking sheet instead.

Tropical Smoothie

CALORIES PER SERVING: 76

Serves 1 │ Preparation time: 5 minutes

This effortlessly easy smoothie will give you a boost at any time of day. The cinnamon gives it an extra layer of flavor, which contrasts with the sweetness of the mango. Try it with other fruits for endless combinations.

½ mango, peeled and
    pitted
1 apple, unpeeled
juice of ½ lime
a pinch of cinnamon

Roughly chop the fruit and put it in a blender with the lime juice, cinnamon and 3 tbsp (50ml) water.

Blend until smooth, then pour into a glass and enjoy!

Citrus Poached Pears

CALORIES PER SERVING: 90

Serves 4 │ Preparation time: 5 minutes │ Cooking time: 40 minutes

The star anise in this light, fruity snack provides an exotic flavor and enhances the sweetness of the pears and honey. This dish can double as a refreshing dessert.

4 pears, peeled
zest and juice of 2
    oranges
zest and juice of 1 lemon
2 tsp honey
1 cinnamon stick
1 star anise

Place the pears in a pan with the orange juice, lemon, honey, cinnamon and star anise. Add ¾c (200ml) water and cover with a circle of parchment paper. Put the lid on the pan and bring to a boil then turn down the heat and simmer for 20–30 minutes, until the pears are tender.

Remove the pears from the liquid and set aside. Bring the mixture to a boil and simmer for a few minutes to reduce to about ⅓c (100ml). Serve each pear with the juice drizzled over.

Biscotti

CALORIES PER BISCOTTI: 90

Makes 50 | Preparation time: 25 minutes | Cooking time: 45 minutes

These light, crunchy biscotti, studded with toasted almonds and with a hint of orange are irresistible. They will keep in an airtight jar for a couple of weeks.

6oz (175g) whole blanched almonds

1 tbsp coriander seeds

½c (125g) unsalted butter, softened

½c (200g) granulated sugar

2 medium eggs, beaten

finely grated zest of 1 orange

1 tbsp Grand Marnier or other orange liqueur

1½ tsp baking powder

½ tsp salt

2¾c (350g) all-purpose flour

2.5oz (75g) coarse-grain polenta (regular or quick-cook)

Preheat the oven to 325°F/170°C. Spread the almonds on a baking sheet and toast in the oven for 5–10 minutes until golden. Allow to cool. Coarsely chop one third of the toasted nuts and mix with the whole ones. Lightly crush the coriander seeds.

In a bowl, cream the butter with the sugar until just mixed. Beat in the eggs, orange zest, liqueur, baking powder and salt. Stir in 2¼c (275g) of the flour, the polenta, almonds and crushed coriander.

Turn the dough onto a floured work surface and knead until smooth, adding the remaining flour little by little, until the dough is soft but not sticky. It may not be necessary to add all of the flour.

Divide the dough into four equal pieces and roll each into a 2in (5cm) wide, ¾in (2cm) deep sausage. Place these on 2 greased baking sheets and bake for about 35 minutes, until just golden around the edges.

Carefully transfer to a wire rack. Allow to cool for 10 minutes, then cut diagonally into ½in (1cm) thick slices. Place these slices, cut-side down, on the baking sheets and bake for another
10 minutes until golden brown. Transfer to a wire rack to cool completely.

Note: Polenta is maize meal and can be bought in different grades. Use coarse meal for biscotti.

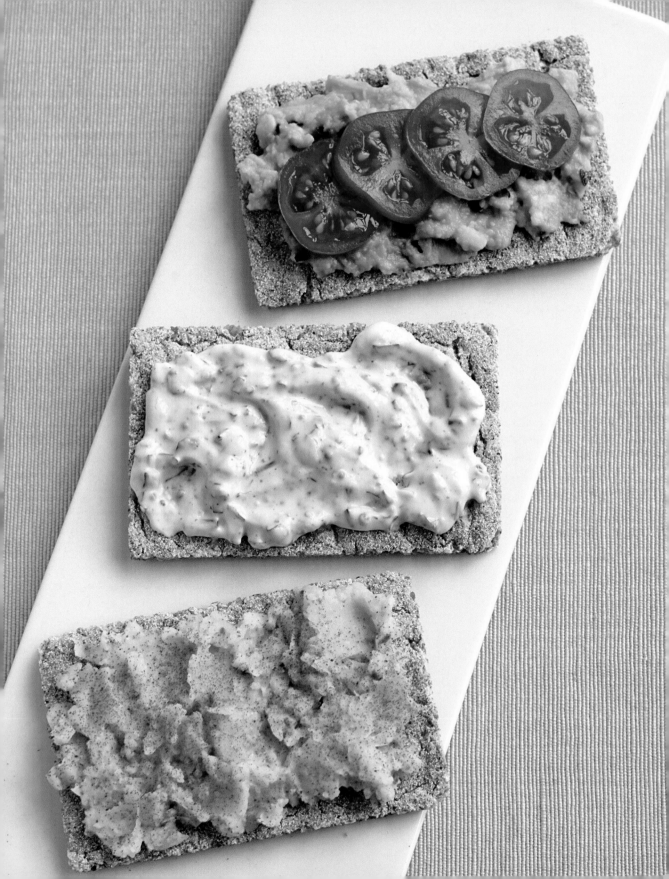

Cracker Toppings

Serves 1

Each of these delicious toppings can be spread liberally on a cracker. The individual calorie counts include the crackers. Alternatively, use them as dips for crunchy vegetables, like carrots and celery.

Spicy Avocado

CALORIES PER SERVING: 100

Preparation time: 5 minutes

Mash a quarter of an avocado with a squeeze of lime and a pinch of chili flakes. Season well with salt and pepper, then spoon on to a cracker and top with sliced tomato.

Herb and Mustard Spread

CALORIES PER SERVING: 75

Preparation time: 5 minutes

Put 0.75oz (20g) low-fat cream cheese in a bowl and beat in 1 teaspoon of grainy mustard and 1 tablespoon of freshly chopped herbs (a mixture of parsley, chives and thyme is ideal) and a squeeze of lemon. Season and mix again, then spoon on to the cracker.

Lima Bean Hummus

CALORIES PER SERVING: 98

Preparation time: 3 minutes

Drain a 14oz (400g) can of lima beans and process in a blender with the juice of 1 lemon and 1 teaspoon each of ground cumin and coriander seeds. Season well with salt and pepper and top 2 crackers with 2 tablespoons of hummus each, and sprinkle with paprika. Keep the rest of the hummus in the fridge, covered; it will last for a couple of days.

Hot and Sour Soup

CALORIES PER SERVING: 100

Serves 2 | Preparation time: 15 minutes | Cooking time: 25 minutes

Look out for packs of Thai mixed spices in larger supermarkets. Each pack usually contains a piece of lemongrass, some Kaffir lime leaves, a couple of hot chilies and a few pieces of kuchai (garlic chives). If you are unable to find a ready-made pack, buy each of these ingredients separately.

1 x packet of fresh Thai mixed spices (see above)

2 garlic cloves, finely sliced

1in (2.5cm) piece fresh ginger root, finely sliced

a handful of cilantro

5c (1.2 liters) chicken stock

1 x 5.25oz (150g) skinless chicken breast fillet

4.5oz (125g) mushrooms, preferably shiitake or baby button mushrooms

1–2 spring onions, to garnish

juice of 2 limes

2 tbsp light soy sauce

Prepare the herbs by crushing the lemongrass using a rolling pin. Finely slice the chilies (retaining the seeds). Put the Thai herbs in a large saucepan along with the garlic, ginger, half the cilantro and the stock. Cover and bring to a boil.

Meanwhile, cut the chicken into strips and halve or slice any larger mushrooms. When the stock has come to a boil, reduce the heat so that it is just simmering. Drop the chicken and mushrooms into the soup. Cover and simmer gently for 20 minutes.

Meanwhile, trim the spring onions and cut into 3in (7.5cm) lengths. Halve each piece lengthways, then cut into very fine shreds. Drop them into a bowl of cold water and leave in the refrigerator to curl. (If you're short on time, you could simply trim the spring onions and cut into thin slices on the diagonal).

Check that the chicken is cooked. Add the lime juice and soy sauce to the soup, then taste. The flavor should be fairly hot and faintly sour. If it needs more salt, add a little extra soy sauce. Remove and discard the cilantro.

Drain the curled spring onion shreds. Ladle the soup into warmed individual bowls and top each with a pile of onion shreds and the rest of the fresh cilantro.

Saffron Scones

CALORIES PER SERVING: 110

Makes 12 | Preparation time: 15 minutes, plus infusing time | Cooking time: 10 minutes

With its golden color, wonderful aroma and intriguing taste, regal saffron gives an exciting lift to the humble scone. These scones can be frozen.

1 tsp saffron threads
⅔c (150ml) milk
2c (225g) self-rising
    white flour
a pinch of salt
1 tsp baking powder
3 tbsp (40g) unsalted
    butter or margarine
2 tbsp baker's sugar
1 medium egg, beaten,
    to glaze

Preheat the oven to 425˚F/220˚C. Lightly grease a baking sheet.

Roughly break up the saffron threads and place in a saucepan with half of the milk. Bring just to a boil, then remove from the heat and leave to infuse for 20 minutes.

Sift the flour, salt and baking powder into a bowl. Add the butter, cut into small pieces, and rub in using your fingertips, until the mixture resembles fine breadcrumbs. Stir in the sugar.

Stir in the saffron milk and half of the remaining milk. Mix with a pastry cutter to create a soft dough, adding the rest of the milk if the mixture is too dry; it should be soft and slightly sticky.

Knead lightly and roll out to a ¾in (2cm) thickness. Cut out rounds, using a 2in (5cm) cutter. Place on the baking sheet and brush the tops with the beaten egg. Bake for 10–12 minutes until well risen and golden brown. Transfer to a wire rack to cool.

Oaty Fruit Bites

CALORIES PER BITE: 113

Makes 16 │ Preparation time: 10 minutes │ Cooking time: 20 minutes

The oats will provide slow-release energy to help keep you full. These freeze really well so wrap up any that you aren't going to eat in plastic wrap and freeze them for up to a month.

3½ tbsp (75g) honey

2 medium eggs

1c (125g) self-rising whole wheat flour

½c less 1 tbsp (75g) oats

2.5oz (75g) golden raisins

1oz (20g) slivered almonds

3½ tbsp (50g) butter, melted

⅓c (75ml) milk

1 tsp pumpkin pie spice

zest of 1 orange

Preheat the oven to 400°F/200°C. Line a shallow 7in (17cm)-square baking pan with parchment paper.

Beat the honey and eggs together in a bowl. Sift in the flour, then add the rest of the ingredients and fold together with a large metal spoon. Spoon into the prepared pan, spread out evenly and bake for 20 minutes.

Using the edges of the parchment paper, lift out the bake and transfer to a wire rack. Leave to cool then cut into 16 squares.

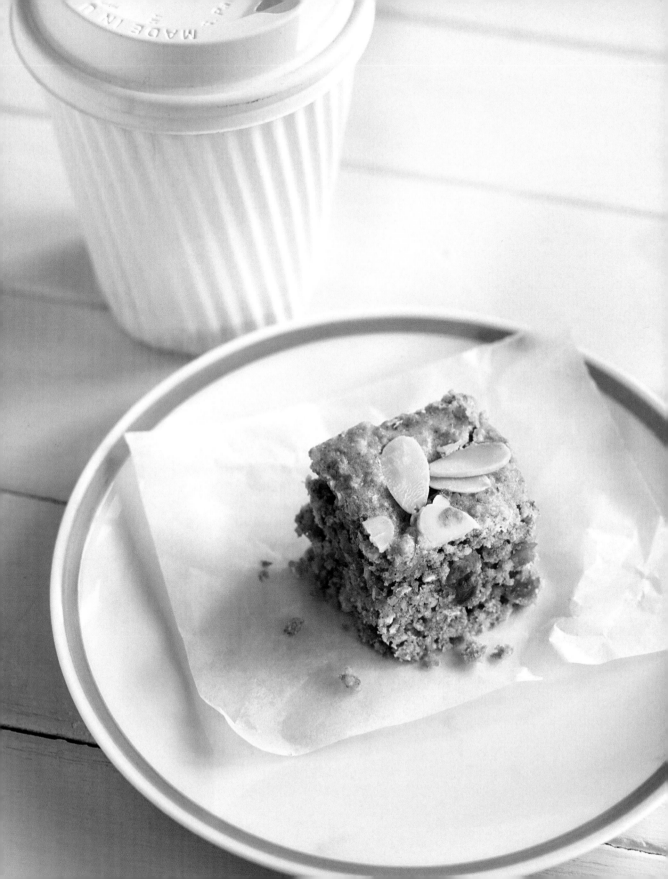

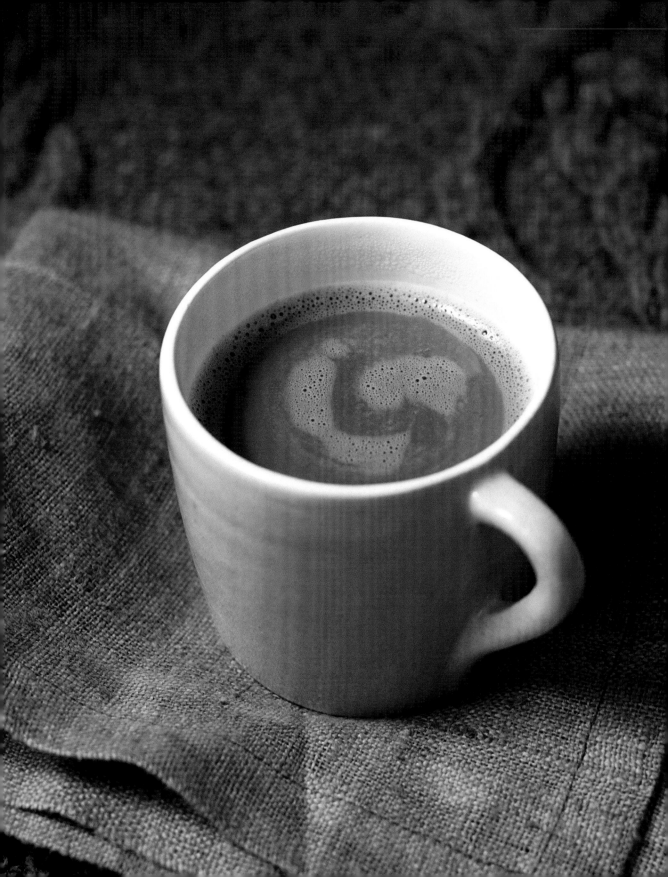

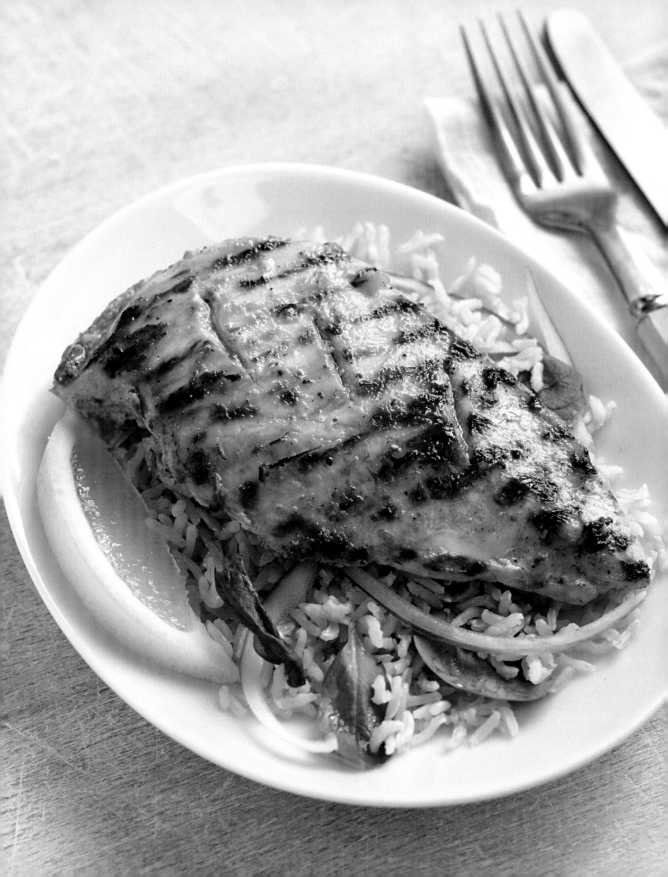

Rich and Dark Spiced Hot Chocolate

CALORIES PER SERVING: 114

Serves 1 | Preparation time: 2 minutes | Cooking time: 5 minutes

Sometimes only chocolate is the answer. This lightly spiced chocolate drink is rich and indulgent and miraculously low in calories.

⅓c (100ml) low-fat milk
3 tbsp (50ml) water
0.5oz (10g) dark
    chocolate (70
    percent cocoa
    solids), grated
1 tsp cocoa powder
½ tsp sugar
1 star anise
a good pinch of
    pumpkin pie spice
¼ vanilla pod

Pour the milk and water into a pan and add the chocolate, cocoa powder, sugar, star anise and pumpkin pie spice. Split the piece of vanilla pod lengthways and scrape the seeds into the liquid. Add the pod too.

Place the pan over medium heat and bring to a boil, whisking all the time to dissolve the chocolate in the liquid. As soon as the mixture is boiling, strain into a cup and serve.

Green Apple Sorbet

118

CALORIES PER SERVING: 118

Serves 4 | Preparation time: 25 minutes, plus chilling and freezing time |
Cooking time: 10 minutes

Make this fresh, summery sorbet with sweet but sharp Granny Smith apples—taste
one to make sure they're sharp enough. The apple brandy provides an extra richness,
but feel free to leave it out if you prefer.

1lb (450g) Granny
    Smith apples
¼c (50g) baker's sugar
2 tbsp lemon or lime
    juice
3 tbsp apple brandy
1 medium egg white,
    lightly beaten

Peel, halve and core the apples. Place in a saucepan with
the sugar and lemon or lime juice. Cover and simmer for
5–10 minutes until tender.

Purée the soft apple mixture in a blender or food processor,
then sieve to remove any lumps. Cool, chill, then stir in the
apple brandy. Churn in an ice-cream maker according to the
manufacturer's instructions, adding the beaten egg white
halfway through freezing.

If you do not have an ice-cream maker, transfer to a shallow
container and freeze for 2 hours. Remove from the freezer
and beat well to break down any ice crystals that may have
formed. Return to the freezer for another hour, then beat
again. Repeat once more. Freeze for several hours, and just
before the sorbet is almost firm, stir in the egg white. Freeze
again until required.

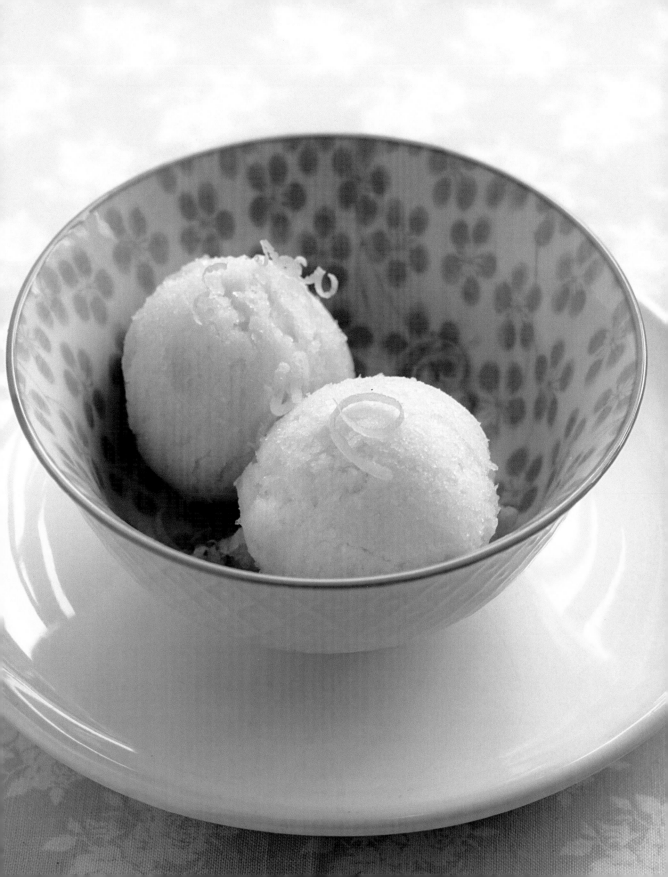

Fruit Salad

CALORIES PER SERVING: 125

Serves 6 | Preparation time: 20 minutes, plus infusing and chilling time | Cooking time: 5 minutes

This refreshing fruit salad is enhanced with a cardamom and mint syrup. Choose ripe fruit in optimum condition. Pineapples should have a rich golden brown skin and a sweet aroma; mangoes should give slightly when gently pressed.

¼c (50g) baker's sugar
4 green cardamom
    pods
6 large mint sprigs
finely grated zest and
    juice of 1 lime
1 medium pineapple
1 large mango
3 small juicy oranges
1 medium papaya

Put the sugar in a small heavy-based pan with ¾c (200ml) water. Crush the cardamom with a rolling pin to split the pods slightly. Crush 4 mint sprigs in the same way. Add the crushed mint and cardamom to the pan.

Heat the mixture gently until the sugar dissolves, then bring to a boil and boil for 1 minute. Allow to cool and infuse for at least 1 hour or until completely cold. Discard the mint sprigs and cardamom pods.

Strip the leaves from the remaining mint sprigs and add them to the sugar syrup with the lime zest and juice. Pour into a bowl and chill while preparing the fruit.

Peel the pineapple, halve and discard the tough central core. Cut the flesh into large chunks. Cut the mango across either side of the pit, then cut the flesh into large slices and peel off the skin. Chop the flesh surrounding the pit. Peel the oranges, then cut each one into wedges. Cut the papaya in half and scoop out the seeds with a teaspoon. Cut the flesh into slices and remove the skin.

Arrange the fruit in a shallow serving dish and pour the syrup on top. Cover the bowl and chill in the refrigerator for 30 minutes before serving.

Note: Don't cut the fruit up too small; keep the pieces chunky and attractive.

Mango, Ginger and Citrus Sorbet

CALORIES PER SERVING: 130

Serves 4 | Preparation time: 25 minutes, plus freezing time | Cooking time: 4 minutes

Mangoes are ideal for making sorbets as their creamy texture lends itself perfectly to the freezing process. The sweetness of the ginger and mango is balanced by the lime juice to produce a tangy, refreshing snack.

2 x 14oz (400g)
    mangoes
1oz (25g) preserved
    stem ginger, drained
50ml syrup from the
    stem ginger jar
¼c (40g) baker's sugar
finely grated zest and
    juice of 3 limes

Peel the mangoes, using a potato peeler, then cut down either side of the central pit; cut away as much of the remaining flesh as possible. Chop the mango flesh and purée in a blender or food processor until very smooth. Transfer to a bowl and set aside. Finely chop the stem ginger and stir into the purée.

Place the ginger syrup in a small pan with the sugar, lime zest and juice, and add ⅓c (90ml) water. Heat gently, stirring until the sugar has dissolved. Bring to a boil and simmer for 3 minutes. Remove from the heat and leave to cool.

Strain the cooled syrup through a fine sieve into the puréed mango mixture and stir well. Transfer to a plastic container and freeze for 2 hours.

Remove from the freezer and beat well to break down any ice crystals that may have formed. Return to the freezer for another hour, then beat again. Repeat once more. Freeze for several hours until firm, or until required. Transfer the sorbet to the refrigerator about 20 minutes before serving to soften slightly. Scoop into individual glass dishes to serve.

Almond Fudge Crumbles

CALORIES PER BISCUIT: 130

Makes 20 | Preparation time: 10 minutes | Cooking time: 12 minutes

At times the only answer is a nibble of something sweet. Hidden pieces of crushed almond slivers and chewy fudge marry perfectly in these simple cookies. This recipe makes enough dough for 20 cookies, so use half and then freeze the other half for up to a month.

1⅔c (200g) all-purpose flour
a pinch of salt
½ tsp baking soda
½c plus 2 tbsp (125g) unsalted butter
½c (125g) muscovado sugar
1 medium egg
1 tsp almond extract
2.5oz (75g) slivered almonds, crumbled
2oz (50g) vanilla fudge, finely diced
powdered sugar, for dusting

Preheat the oven to 375˚F/190˚C. Lightly grease two baking sheets.

Sift the flour, salt and baking soda into a bowl. Add the butter, cut into small pieces, and rub in using your fingertips.

Add the sugar, egg, almond extract, ⅓c (65g) of the slivered almonds and 1.5oz (40g) of the fudge and mix to form a fairly firm dough.

Turn on to a lightly floured surface and roll into a cylinder about 9in (23cm) long. (At this point you can freeze any of the dough you're not planning on using.) Cut the dough into rounds and arrange them on the prepared baking sheets, leaving a little space between each one.

Scatter over the remaining almonds and fudge and press down lightly. Bake the cookies for 12 minutes, until turning golden around the edges. Leave on the baking sheets for 5 minutes, then transfer to a wire rack to cool. Serve dusted with powdered sugar.

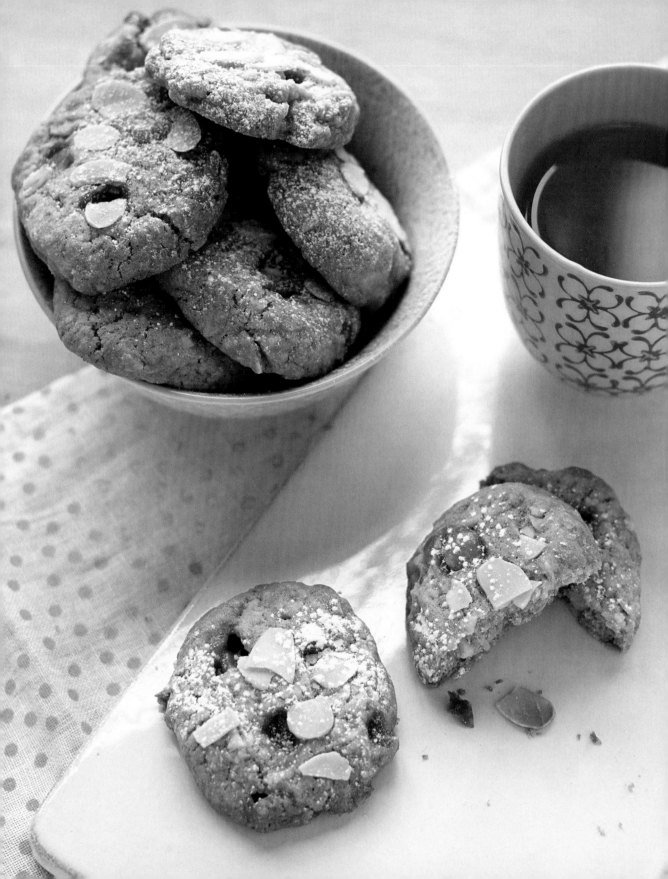

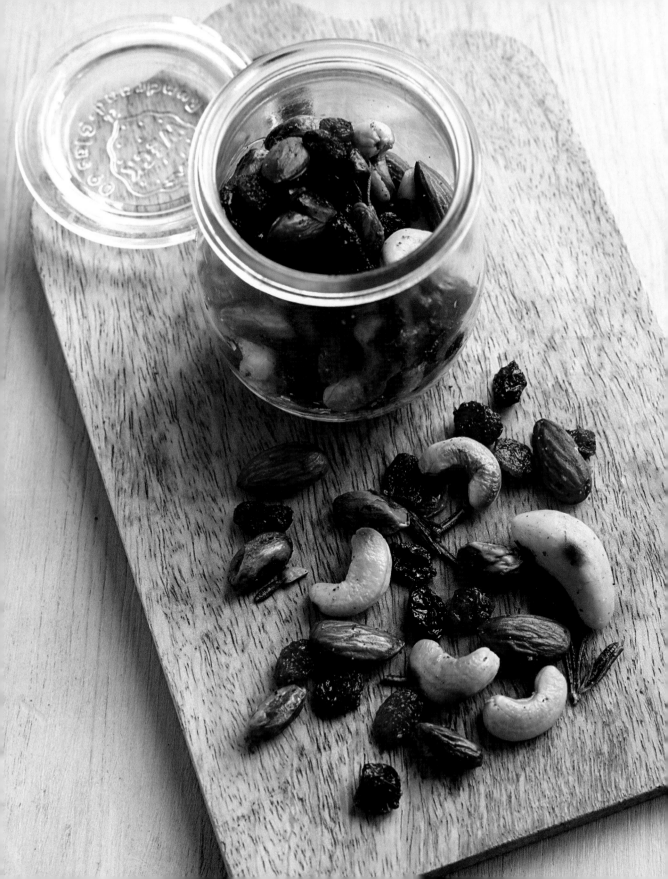

Spicy Trail Mix

CALORIES PER SERVING: 154

Makes 10 x 30g servings | Preparation time: 5 minutes | Cooking time: 15 minutes

Crunchy and spicy, this nutty mix will stave off midafternoon hunger pangs. Keep a portion in your bag for when you're out and about and store the rest in an airtight jar, where it will keep for about a week.

2oz (50g) pistachio
   nuts
2oz (50g) Brazil nuts
2oz (50g) almonds
2oz (50g) cashews
1 tsp olive oil
½ tsp garlic granules
1 tsp cayenne pepper
1 tsp chopped rosemary
   leaves
2oz (50g) golden raisins
2oz (50g) dried
   cranberries

Preheat the oven to 400˚F/200˚C. Put the nuts in a roasting pan and drizzle over the oil. Add the garlic, cayenne and rosemary and mix everything together. Make sure the nuts are coated in the oil.

Roast in the oven for 10 minutes then add the golden raisins and cranberries and continue to roast for another 5 minutes.

Remove from the oven and leave to cool slightly. Store in an airtight jar for up to a week.

Individual Summer Bread Puddings

160

CALORIES PER SERVING: 160

Serves 6 | Preparation time: 30 minutes, plus chilling time | Cooking time: 12 minutes

An old favorite, individual summer bread puddings are ideal to serve as part of a healthy diet, especially if you use whole wheat bread. Fruit of any description is good to use here— summer puddings can be made into autumn puddings by using apples, pears and plums.

12 large slices of whole
    wheat bread, crusts
    removed
10oz (300g)
    blackberries
14oz (400g) raspberries
4.5oz (125g) cranberries
6oz (175g) Concord
    grapes
⅔c (150ml) red grape
    juice
2 tbsp chopped mint
artificial sweetener, to
    taste

Line six muffin cups in a muffin pan with plastic wrap. Cut a 2in (5cm) circle of bread to fit the base of each cup. Cut six 3in (7.5cm) circles of bread and set aside. Cut the remaining bread into strips and use to line the sides of the cups completely.

Wash and pat dry the blackberries, raspberries, cranberries and grapes.

Place the cranberries in a saucepan with the grape juice, cover and cook for 5 minutes. Add the remaining fruit and cook gently for 5–7 minutes. Stir the mint into the fruit and add sweetener, to taste.

While the fruit is still warm, spoon into the lined muffin cups, using a slotted spoon, and pour on sufficient fruit juice to moisten. Reserve the rest of the fruit juice. Cover with the reserved bread rounds. Top each cup with a saucer or plate and press down with a heavy weight. Place in the fridge for several hours or overnight.

Turn out the puddings on to serving plates and pour on the reserved juice to cover them.

Spiced Baked Apple

CALORIES PER SERVING: 163

Serves 1 | Preparation time: 10 minutes | Cooking time: 45–50 minutes

A sweet and filling snack that you could even serve as a dessert. You could use another type of apple, but Granny Smiths are ideal because they hold their shape as they cook.

1 Granny Smith apple
1 ready-to-eat dried
    apricot, finely
    chopped
1 dried date, finely
    chopped
4 whole almonds, finely
    chopped
½ tsp pumpkin pie spice
½ tsp honey
juice of ½ orange
1 slightly heaped tbsp
    fat-free Greek-style
    yogurt

Preheat the oven to 400°F/200°C.

Core the apple and use a sharp knife to cut the skin around the equator—this stops the apple from exploding during baking.

Mix together the chopped apricot, date, almonds, pumpkin pie spice, honey and orange juice.

Place the apple in a small ovenproof dish and spoon the fruit mixture into the cavity of the apple. Pour enough boiling water into the dish to just cover the base, then cover the whole dish with foil. Bake for 45–50 minutes, until the apple is soft. Serve with the yogurt.

Egg "Mayo" on Rye

CALORIES PER SERVING: 190

Serves 1 | Preparation time: 10 minutes | Cooking time: 10 minutes

Eggs are powerhouses of nutrition and will keep you feeling full for hours. Try this light mayo-style dressing and serve on a slice of dark rye bread. The pea shoots will provide a satisfying, fresh crunch.

1 medium egg
1 tsp olive oil
1 tsp Dijon mustard
a squeeze of lemon
    juice
1 tbsp chopped
    peppercress
½ slice dark rye bread
    (1oz/30g)
salt and pepper
a handful of watercress
    or pea shoots, to
    serve

Place the egg in a pan of water and bring to a boil. Simmer for 7 minutes. Lift the cooked egg out of the pan and hold under cold running water to cool quickly.

Remove the shell from the egg. Using a fork, roughly crush the egg in a bowl.

Whisk together the oil, mustard and lemon juice and season well. Add to the egg along with the chopped peppercress and fold everything together.

Spoon on top of the rye bread and top with the watercress or pea shoots.

Pickled Salmon on Rye

CALORIES PER SERVING: 199

Serves 2 | Preparation time: 25 minutes, plus resting and chilling time

This homemade gravlax incorporates a dash of teriyaki marinade and a little fresh ginger to give it a Japanese overtone. Slice it vertically and very finely and serve on dark rye bread. The pickled salmon keeps well in the fridge.

4.5oz (125g) salmon, filleted and trimmed, but not skinned
¼ tsp vegetable oil
¼in (0.5cm) piece fresh ginger root
1 tsp sugar
1 tsp coarse sea salt
1 tsp white peppercorns, crushed
½ tbsp vodka or rice wine (saki)
1 tsp teriyaki marinade
2 thin slices of dark rye bread
2oz (50g) salad greens
½ tsp chopped chives, to garnish

for the sauce
1 tbsp horseradish (or milder creamed horseradish)
¼in (0.5cm) piece fresh ginger root

Remove any small bones from the salmon with tweezers. Rub the flesh with the oil. Peel and finely chop the ginger and mix with the sugar, salt and crushed peppercorns.

Put the salmon fillet, skin-side down, on a large sheet of parchment paper on top of a sheet of foil. Spread the spice mixture evenly over the flesh. Moisten with the vodka and teriyaki marinade. Wrap up tightly in the paper and then the foil. Place in a non-corrosive dish and cover with a small plate. Place a 1lb (450g) weight on top and leave at cool room temperature for 4 hours.

After 4 hours, turn the packet over and replace the plate and weight. Leave for another 4 hours, then remove the weight and refrigerate for 4 hours. The salmon is ready to eat, but the longer it sits in the marinade, the stronger the flavor will become.

For the sauce, put the horseradish in a small bowl. Peel and chop the ginger and squeeze through a garlic press into the horseradish, and mix to combine.

Unwrap the salmon packet, retaining the juices, and scrape off the excess peppercorns. Slice the salmon vertically, into ¼in (0.5cm)-thick slices, then cut horizontally, close to the skin, to release each slice.

Spread a little sauce on each slice of rye bread. Arrange the pickled salmon slices on the bread. Serve with a little salad, a drizzle of marinade and a sprinkling of chives.

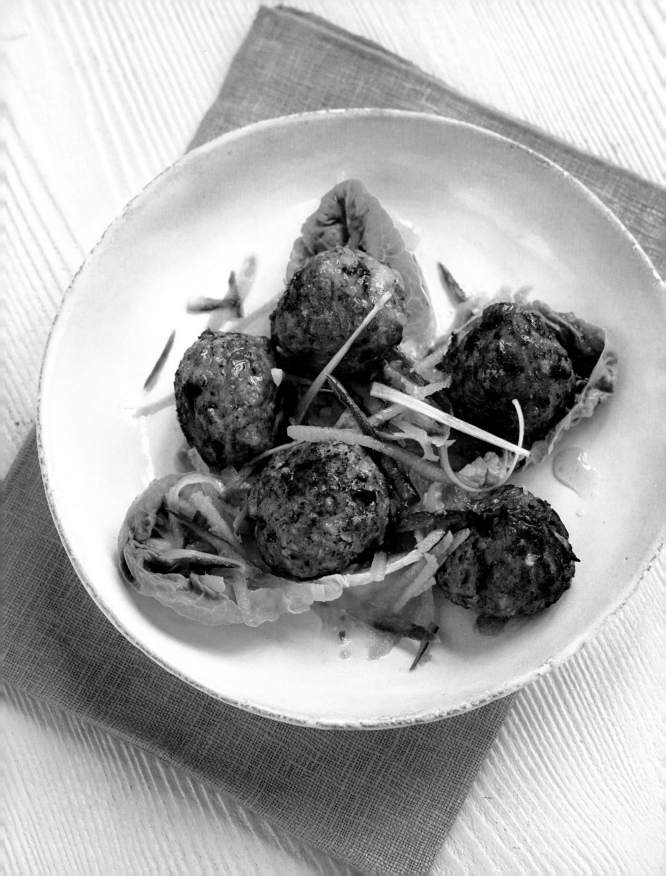

Spiced Pork Balls with Sweet Chili Sauce

CALORIES PER SERVING: 200 (39 calories per pork ball)

Makes 20 balls │ Preparation time: 10 minutes │ Cooking time: 10 minutes

These hearty little meaty snacks are deliciously spicy, and don't seem like a low-calorie option at all. Served with the chile sauce dip and a crisp salad, they make a very satisfying snack, or could even be served as a light lunch or dinner.

1in (2.5cm) piece fresh
    ginger root, peeled
    and halved
2 garlic cloves, peeled
2 shallots, peeled and
    quartered
2 red chiles
1 tsp Chinese five spice
6 tbsp chopped cilantro
18oz (500g) pork fillet,
    roughly chopped
1 medium egg, beaten
a little plain flour, for
    rolling
2 tsp vegetable oil
12 Little Gem lettuce
    leaves
salt and white pepper
4 spring onions,
    shredded, to garnish

for the sauce
2 tbsp sweet chili sauce
1 tbsp rice wine vinegar
½ small carrot, coarsely
    grated
⅛ cucumber, grated

Place the ginger, garlic, shallots and chiles (remove the seeds if you don't like it too hot) in a food processor or blender and process until finely chopped.

Add the five spice, cilantro, pork and egg. Process again until evenly mixed. Season with the salt and white pepper.

Using lightly floured hands, shape the mixture into 20 walnut-sized balls.

Heat a little oil in a non-stick frying pan and fry the balls, in batches, on each side until golden and cooked through.

In a small bowl, stir together the sweet chili sauce, vinegar, carrot and cucumber. Divide the Little Gem lettuce leaves between four plates, top with the balls, drizzle with the sauce and serve garnished with shredded spring onions.

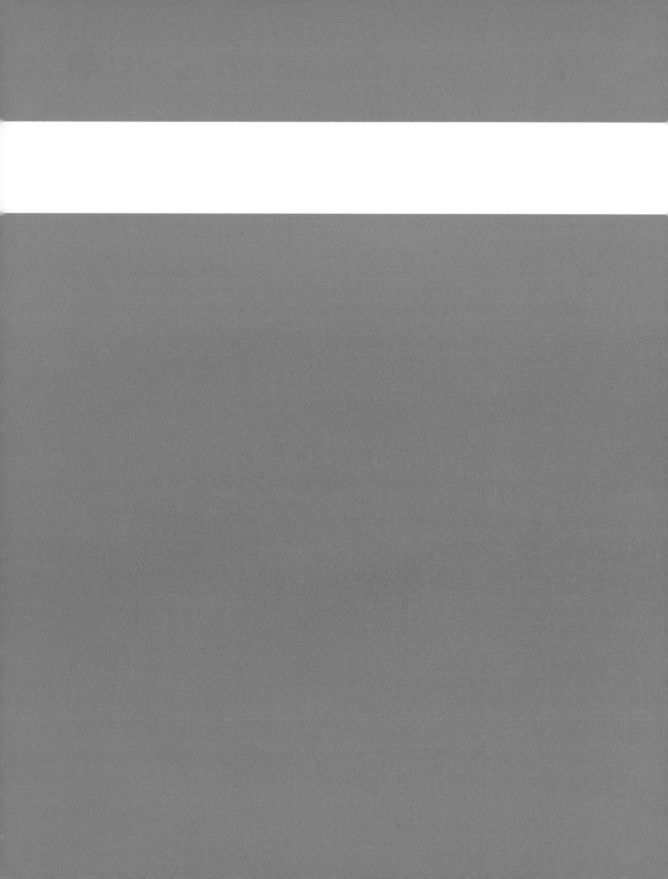

meal plans

Day 1

TOTAL CALORIES PER SERVING: 481

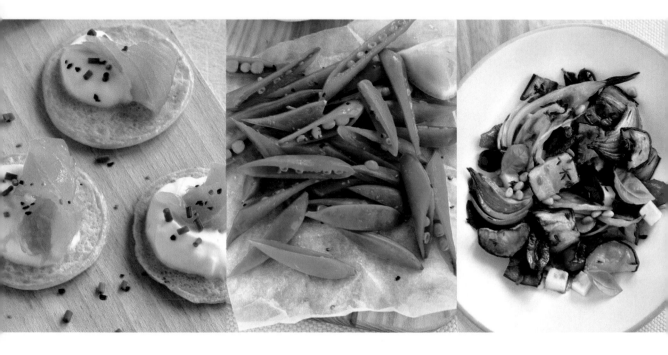

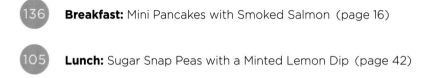

136   **Breakfast:** Mini Pancakes with Smoked Salmon   (page 16)

105   **Lunch:** Sugar Snap Peas with a Minted Lemon Dip   (page 42)

240   **Dinner:** Warm Roasted Vegetable Salad   (page 121)

Day 2

497

TOTAL CALORIES PER SERVING: 497

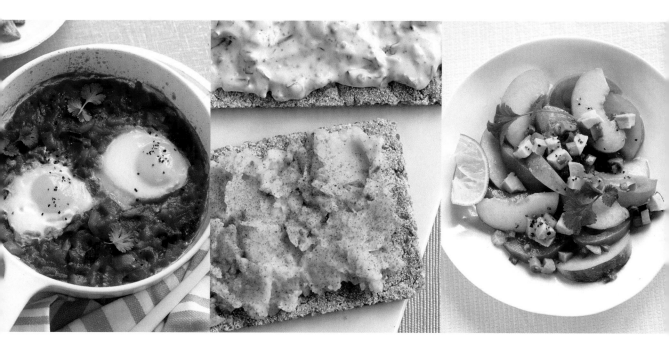

204 **Breakfast:** Huevos Rancheros (page 22)

98 **Snack:** Lima Bean Hummus on Crackers (page 157)

195 **Dinner:** Tomato and Peach Salad with Avocado Salsa (page 111)

Day 3

TOTAL CALORIES PER SERVING: 508

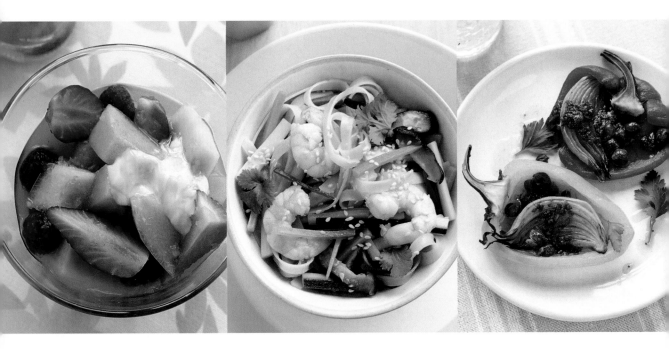

112 **Breakfast:** Melon with Summer Fruits (page 13)

171 **Lunch:** Prawn and Rice Noodle Salad (page 49)

135 **Dinner:** Grilled Stuffed Peppers (page 98)

90 **Snack:** Biscotti (page 155)

Day 4

TOTAL CALORIES PER SERVING: 518

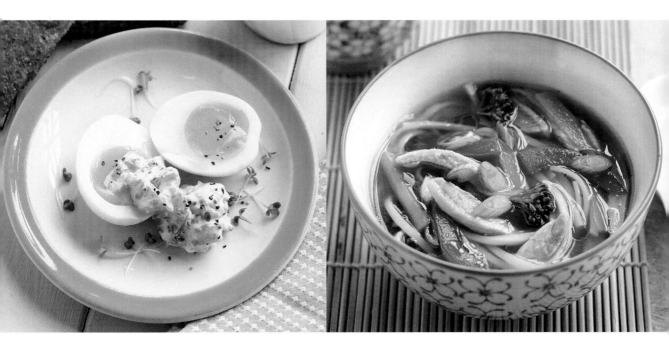

249 **Breakfast:** Eggs with Smoked Salmon (page 29)

229 **Lunch:** Asian-Style Chicken Noodle Soup (page 60)

40 **Snack:** Koftas (page 152)

Day 5

TOTAL CALORIES PER SERVING: 528

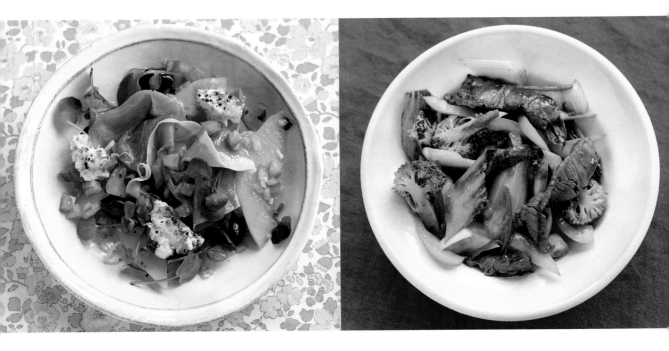

228 **Breakfast:** Prosciutto, Melon and Ricotta Salad (page 26)

100 **Lunch:** Mushroom Pâté with Madeira (page 40)

200 **Dinner:** Chinese Beef (page 114)

Day 6

TOTAL CALORIES PER SERVING: 538

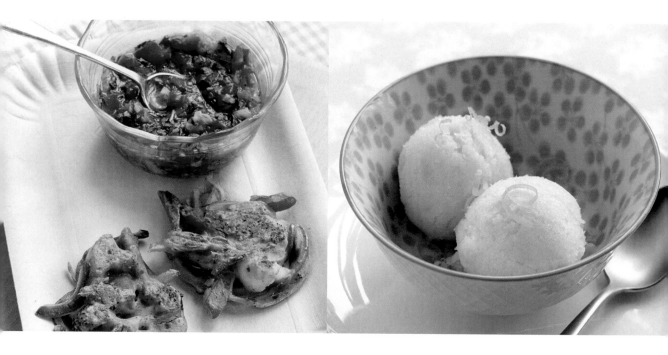

105 **Breakfast:** Chilled Melon and Ginger Salad (page 12)

215 **Lunch:** Indian Spiced Fritters with Cilantro Chutney (page 59)

100 **Dinner:** Thai Fishcakes (page 96)

118 **Snack:** Green Apple Sorbet (page 164)

Day 7

555

TOTAL CALORIES PER SERVING: 555

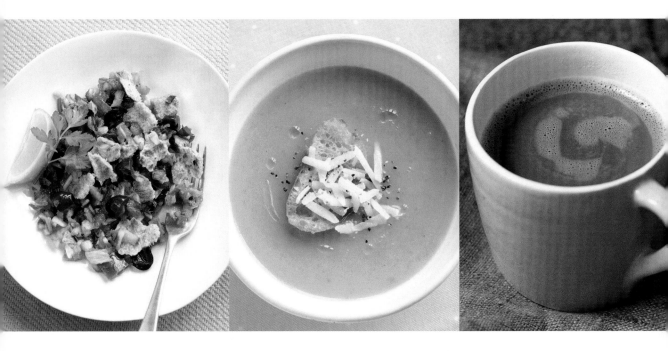

76 **Snack:** Tropical Smoothie (page 154)

180 **Lunch:** Fattoush (page 53)

185 **Dinner**: Butternut Squash Soup with Parmesan Crostini (page 108)

114 **Snack:** Rich and Dark Spiced Hot Chocolate (page 163)

186 | meal plans

Day 8

570

TOTAL CALORIES PER SERVING: 570

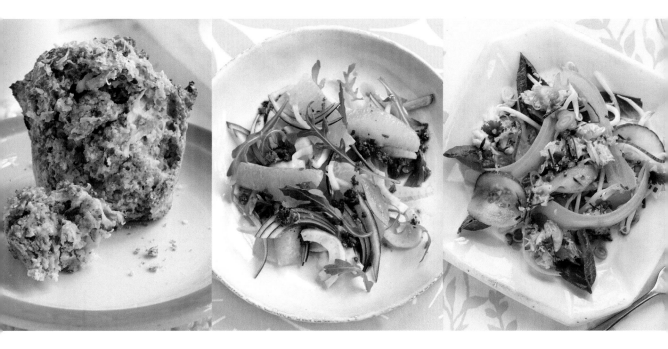

215 **Breakfast:** Savory Muffins (page 25)

185 **Lunch:** Fennel and Orange Salad (page 54)

170 **Dinner:** Crab Salad (page 105)

index

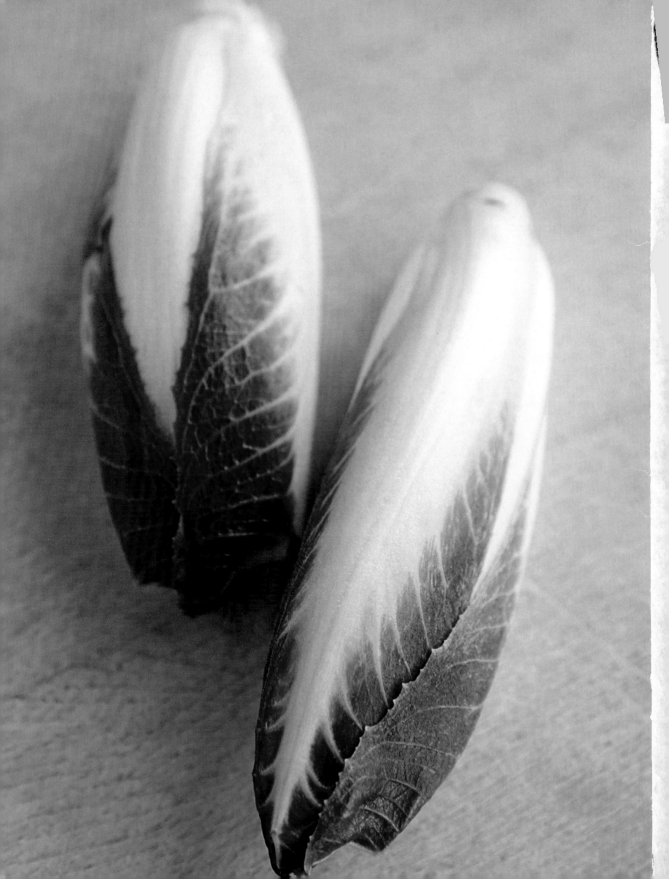

Paella

CALORIES PER SERVING: 405

Serves 6 | Preparation time: 30 minutes | Cooking time: 40 minutes

Paella, a traditional Spanish dish, is a typical example of the good balance of food found in the Mediterranean diet. A colorful all-in-one dish, it is excellent for an informal supper.

2 x 5.25oz (150g) skinless chicken breasts
2 tbsp olive oil
8oz (225g) cleaned and prepared squid
4.5oz (125g) scallops
8oz (225g) live mussels in shells
1 large onion
8oz (225g) plum tomatoes
3 garlic cloves, crushed
1 tsp paprika
2½c (600ml) chicken stock
1 tbsp tomato purée
12oz (350g) Arborio rice
5oz (150ml) dry white wine
a pinch of saffron threads
2 red peppers
4.5oz (125g) shelled peas
2 tbsp chopped flat-leaf parsley
salt and pepper

Cut each chicken breast crosswise into 4 pieces. Heat 1 tablespoon of the oil in a paella pan, large non-stick frying pan or Dutch oven. Toss the chicken pieces quickly in the oil to brown. Remove and set aside.

Cut off the tentacles and slice the squid into thin rings. Slice each scallop into 2 or 3 rounds, depending on their thickness. Set both aside.

Wash the mussels thoroughly in plenty of cold water, scrubbing well, and remove the beards. Discard any which do not close when tapped firmly. Place in a large pan with about 6 tablespoons of water. Bring to a boil, then cover tightly and cook for 3–4 minutes until the shells have opened; discard any that do not open. Set aside.

Finely chop the onion. Immerse the tomatoes in a bowl of boiling water for 30 seconds. Remove from the water and pull away the skins. Chop the flesh into ½in (1cm) pieces.

Heat the remaining oil in the chicken pan. Add the onion, tomatoes, garlic and paprika, and season with salt and pepper. Stir well and cook gently for 7–10 minutes, until softened.

In another pan, heat the chicken stock to just below boiling point, then stir in the tomato purée.

continued on page 144

Paella cont.

Add the rice to the onion and tomato mixture and cook, stirring, for 1 minute. Pour in 1¼c (300ml) of the hot stock and the wine. Cook, stirring, for about 7 minutes, until the liquid has been absorbed.

Meanwhile, soak the saffron threads in the remaining stock. Add to the rice with the squid, scallops and chicken. Cover and simmer gently for 15 minutes.

Meanwhile, preheat the grill to high and grill the red peppers, turning, until blackened. Cover with a damp towel, leave until cool enough to handle, then remove the skins. Cut the peppers in half, remove the core and seeds, then cut into thin strips.

Stir the peppers into the paella with the mussels, peas and parsley. Cook for another 5 minutes. Check the seasoning and serve immediately.

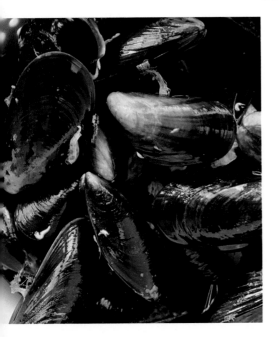

Stir-Fried Jumbo Prawns with Sesame Noodles

CALORIES PER SERVING: 410

Serves 4 | Preparation time: 10 minutes | Cooking time: 10 minutes

Ginger and spring onions give piquancy to the prawns, while soy and sesame add deep flavor to the noodles and vegetables.

2 tsp sesame seeds
1 tsp salt
5.25oz (150g) snow peas,
9oz (250g) dried egg noodles
2 tbsp vegetable oil
16 raw jumbo prawns
4 spring onions, roughly chopped
3in (7.5cm) piece fresh ginger root, grated
juice of 1 lime
2 tsp chopped cilantro leaves
2 tbsp light soy sauce
1 tsp sesame oil
lime wedges, to serve

Put the sesame seeds in a small, heavy-based pan and shake over medium heat until they begin to turn golden and develop a toasted aroma. Tip the toasted sesame seeds out onto a saucer.

Trim the snow peas. Bring a large pan of water to a boil, add the salt and snow peas and return to a boil. Simmer for 30 seconds, then drop in the egg noodles, turn off the heat and leave to stand for 6 minutes.

Meanwhile, heat the oil in a wide frying pan. Add the prawns and cook for 1½–2 minutes on each side, scattering on the spring onions and ginger before you turn them. Squeeze on the lime juice and sprinkle on the cilantro when the prawns are cooked.

Drain the noodles and snow peas and toss in the soy sauce, sesame oil and toasted sesame seeds. Transfer to heated serving plates. Arrange the prawns and spring onions on top and serve with lime wedges.

Steak with Pepper Sauce

CALORIES PER SERVING: 413

Serves 2 | Preparation time: 10 minutes | Cooking time: 40 minutes

A simple steak supper in a rich sauce. Make sure you use beef that has been trimmed of fat.

2 medium sweet
    potatoes, chopped
2 tsp olive oil
1 garlic clove, sliced
4.5oz (125g)
    mushrooms,
    quartered
2 x 5.25oz (150g) pieces
    lean beef fillet
1 tsp roughly crushed
    black peppercorns
3.5oz (100g) green
    beans
3 tbsp (50ml) red wine
⅔c (150ml) hot beef
    stock
1 tsp Concord grape
    jelly
1 tsp butter
2oz (50g) watercress
salt and pepper

Put the sweet potatoes in a pan and cover with cold water. Bring to a boil and simmer for around 15 minutes, until tender. Drain well, then season and mash.

Heat 1 teaspoon of the oil in a pan and add the garlic. Cook for 1 minute. Add the mushrooms, season with salt and pepper, and cover the pan with a lid. Cook for 3–4 minutes, shaking the pan every now and then.

Rub 1 teaspoon of the oil over each piece of beef and press in the crushed peppercorns.

Heat a non-stick frying pan and cook the beef for 3–5 minutes on each side for medium done. Set aside on a warm plate, cover with foil and let rest. Steam the green beans.

Add the red wine, stock and jelly to the frying pan and season with salt and pepper. Bring to a boil and simmer for a few minutes until syrupy. Whisk in the butter.

Divide the mash and green beans between two plates. Place the beef on top, then spoon the mushrooms and sauce on top and serve with a handful of watercress.

Fettucine with Gorgonzola and Spinach

CALORIES PER SERVING: 420

Serves 6 │ Preparation time: 15 minutes │ Cooking time: 10 minutes

The rich and creamy flavor of this pasta sauce belies its few simple ingredients. Use small young, tender spinach leaves if possible.

12oz (350g) baby
   spinach
8oz (225g) Gorgonzola
   cheese
⅓c (75ml) low-fat milk
1½ tbsp (25g) butter
14oz (400g) fresh
   fettucine, tagliatelle
   or long fusilli
salt and pepper
freshly grated nutmeg,
   to serve

Wash the spinach thoroughly and remove any large stalks. Place in a clean saucepan and cook, stirring, over medium-high heat for 2–3 minutes until wilted. There is no need to add extra water—the small amount clinging to the leaves after washing provides sufficient moisture. Drain well in a colander or sieve, pressing out any excess liquid.

Cut the Gorgonzola into small pieces. Place in a clean pan with the milk and butter. Heat gently, stirring, until melted to a creamy sauce. Stir in the drained spinach. Season to taste with pepper; salt may not be necessary because the Gorgonzola is quite salty.

Just before serving, cook the pasta in a large pan of boiling salted water according to packet instructions.

Drain the pasta thoroughly and add to the sauce. Toss well to mix. Serve at once, sprinkled with a little freshly grated nutmeg.

Grilled Chicken with a Spiced Yogurt Crust

CALORIES PER SERVING: 440

Serves 4 │ Preparation time: 10 minutes, plus marinating │ Cooking time: 20 minutes

Yogurt makes a wonderful basis for a marinade, as it tenderizes and adds flavor yet doesn't disappear during cooking. Instead it forms a delicious soft crust, which protects the meat from the fierce heat of the grill.

4 x 4.5oz (125g) skinless chicken breasts
1 tbsp coriander seeds
1 tsp ground cumin
2 tsp mild curry paste
1 garlic clove, crushed
15oz (450ml) Greek-style yogurt
3 tbsp chopped cilantro
7oz (200g) quick-cook brown rice
7oz (200g) spinach leaves
¼ red onion, finely sliced
salt and pepper
1 lemon, cut into wedges, to serve

Slash the chicken breasts two or three times. Crush the coriander seeds, using a pestle and mortar. Mix with the cumin, curry paste, garlic and yogurt in a large shallow dish. Season with salt and pepper and stir in the cilantro.

Add the chicken and turn to coat thoroughly with the spiced yogurt mixture. Leave to marinate for 30 minutes, or cover and place in the fridge overnight.

Preheat the grill to high. Grill the chicken, turning occasionally, for about 20 minutes or until cooked through.

Cook the rice according to the packet instructions. Wash the spinach and cook in a hot pan until just wilted. Toss the rice with the spinach and red onion.

Serve the chicken with the rice and a wedge of lemon to squeeze over.